The Quantum Mind
and Healing

Books by Arnold Mindell

The Quantum Mind and Healing

How to Listen and Respond to Your Body's Symptoms

ARNOLD MINDELL, PH.D.

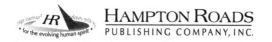

HAMPTON ROADS
PUBLISHING COMPANY, INC.

Cover design by Steve Amarillo
Cover art by Steve Amarillo
Illustrations pgs. 38, 39, and 119 © 2004 by Anne L. Louque.
All rights reserved.

Hampton Roads Publishing Company, Inc.
1125 Stoney Ridge Road
Charlottesville, VA 22902

434-296-2772
fax: 434-296-5096
e-mail: hrpc@hrpub.com
www.hrpub.com

If you are unable to order this book from your local
bookseller, you may order directly from the publisher.
Call 1-800-766-8009, toll-free.

Library of Congress Cataloging-in-Publication Data

Mindell, Arnold, 1940-
   The quantum mind and healing : how to listen and respond to your
body's symptoms : an acclaimed therapist's breakthrough redefines the
mechanics of health / Arnold Mindell.
        p. cm.
Includes bibliographical references.
   ISBN 1-57174-395-2 (alk. paper)
   1. Healing--Miscellanea. 2. Quantum theory. 3. Mind and body. 4.
Consciousness. I. Title.
   RZ999.M543 2004
   615.8'9--dc22
                                        2003025992

ISBN 1-57174-395-2
10 9 8 7 6 5 4 3 2 1
Printed on acid-free paper in the United States

Contents

I. The Force of Silence in Symptoms

   Dreaming is a guiding body force along a given path; if
   ignored, the path is called *dis*-ease.

   New medicine combines alternative and classical theory,
   altered states, and spiritual experience.

   Quantum mechanics and kundalini energy are basic to
   consciousness.

   Mathematical spaces give new insights into symptom
   work.

   With shamanic training, symptoms create surprisingly
   new lifestyles.

II. Nonlocal Medicine: The World in Symptoms

III. Aging: Chemistry, Buddhism, and Entropy

Acknowledgments

Thanks to . . .

Susan Kocen, for transcribing my original lectures and seminars given at the Process Work Center of Portland, Oregon.

Dear participants in my original classes and seminars in Portland, London, Zurich, Tokyo, and many other cities, given with my partner Amy Mindell, on the topics of quantum medicine. Your experimenting, listening, and questioning drew these ideas out of me.

Richard Leviton of Hampton Roads, for your encouraging interest in this book, and for suggesting the first subtitle, "Quantum Dimensions of Symptoms." His ideas released many new thoughts with me.

Margaret Ryan, for your remarkable ability to add to, and bring out, crucial ideas through editing. How do you manage to get inside the author's mind so well?

Carl Mindell, for telling me the original version was too full of physics and helping me relate better to doctors and patients.

Randee Levine Tully, for catching my errors in music.

Sharon Sessions at the physics department of the University of Oregon, for checking my physics, especially thoughts about what thermodynamics says about the universe.

Heiko Spoddeck for helping me with many details, and asking me to be more aware of when I was in an everyday mode of thinking, and when I was thinking as a dreamer.

Dawn Menken, Jan Dworkin, Max Schupbach, Joe Goodbread, and other friends for having steered me toward the endeavor of relating the science of bodywork to the deepest experiences of the mind.

My friends and courageous interpreters and re-creators of physics, Fred Alan Wolf, Nick Herbert, and Amit Goswami for the forerunning nature of your work.

To those who helped me understand medicine and alternative nonlocal medicine, Jai Tomlin, Pierre Morin, Mitch Stargrove, and Larry Dossey.

Dear ghosts of teachers, who sit around me as I write this book: Marie-Louise von Franz, who introduced me to C. G. Jung's idea of synchronicity in Zurich in 1961; Franz Riklin, for introducing me to shamanism and showing me how to live it in everyday life; C. G., for your background support in all things concerning what you called "psyche and matter."

The various allopathic, alternative, and complementary medical doctors who have been my clients, friends, and helpers, for what I have learned from you.

Though they no longer are alive, I must thank the amazing parents of quantum physics, Louis DeBroglie, Erwin Schrödinger, John von Neumann, David Bohm, and Richard Feynman; and the living physicists of hyperspaces, Michio Kaku and Stephen Hawking, for their statements about the virtual spaces, imaginary times, and other realities behind life.

Dear Amy, your work on creativity taught me to take puppets seriously. Together with those puppets, your scientific spirit helped test, clarify, and educate me about the quantum dimensions of symptoms I think no physicist (without a puppet) ever thought of. You helped develop and teach just about every chapter of this work. Thank you.

Preface

How do our thoughts affect our bodies? How do we use our awareness to transform the experience of body symptoms? What can we do to deal with the fear and pain connected to headaches and backaches, lumps and bumps, fatigue and dizziness? What role, if any, does our subjective experience have in cancer or heart trouble? Is it all caused by genetics, the environment, and chance? Is there intelligence behind all these problems?

Yes. There is a deep form of intelligence in the background. I call it the quantum mind and will show how it can be a source of healing.

In *The Quantum Mind and Healing* I explore connections between traditional biomedicine and alternative medical procedures, and suggest experiential and quantum mechanical foundations for the body's intelligence. My therapeutic work with individuals and groups drove me to study special areas of psychology, physics, and medicine to combine these sciences. This book is based upon the discovery of the similar basic patterns underlying our subtlest experiences *and* subatomic physics. The discovery of these patterns has lead me to develop new ways of thinking about people and working with body symptoms.

The study of nano-events and nanomedicine ("nano-" is a prefix meaning the one-billionth part [10^{-9}] of a unit of measurement, here meant to speak of atomic and molecular processes occurring within one-billionth of a meter) will soon create many advances in present-day medicine. Medicine and the associated disciplines of psychology and physics will be drawn together even more than they are today. Yet there are few known unifying paradigms connecting research in anatomy, psychology, psychobiology, biophysics, medical engineering, medical education, general practice, and medical diagnosis with the many psychotherapies, including movement and music therapy.

The first purpose of *The Quantum Mind and Healing* is to focus on body symptoms. This book is meant to be primarily practical. At the same time, a second goal is to suggest unifying ideas bringing together the fields just mentioned. The practice suggested in this book is based on scientific findings and ideas from ancient traditions. I elaborate on these findings and traditions in sidebar discussions throughout. The scientifically minded reader will find additional elaboration of ideas and theories in the appendices.

Writing has brought up numerous feelings in me. In the evening before beginning the final writing of this book, I awoke in a dream. In that dream, I realized I was in the high mountains, in the cool nighttime air. Some grand force had pressed me to hike in the mountains, until I was standing alone on a path, facing a rocky wall, the side of a high, craggy peak. In the shadows of the darkness, I could sense the presence of some kind of mind and an awesome force emanating from the mountainside. I could feel but not describe that force.

Waking up, I suddenly knew the title of this book about body symptoms should be connected to the intelligence and forces of nature, to what I have called the Quantum Mind. In a half-slumber, I wrote the following paragraphs, which felt like a communication from that mountainside force, addressing all of us humans. Today, my everyday mind rebels against these paragraphs because of their self-certain outrageousness.

The direction of your life appears clearly in some dreams. However, in everyday life, you behave as if you are uncertain about what to do next. During the day, you sense a certain but subtle force of silence emanating from the deepest spaces of the night, moving your body into life, and yet, you usually choose to ignore this force.

Looking back over your life, you notice how that force has always been present. In fact, the path of your life seems almost inevitable. What seemed at one time or another to be accidental, upon reflection appears to have been unavoidable. In the moment, life seems chaotic, haphazard. Looking back at your life, however, you see that the force of silence was behind every apparently random act. The specific path you call your "life" seems inevitable, though at given moments in the past you thought you could negotiate with that force. Looking back, the path seems inexorable. Retrospectively you realize that you could only agree with that force and move with it, or disagree and be destroyed.

It is useless pretending this force does not exist, for ignoring its presence turns it into a terrifying event of body symptoms. Act like the force is not here, and life turns sour and space fills with ghosts. Open up to the force of silence in everyday life, and life appears as an infinite, awesome journey.

The force of silence is connected not only with your personal existence, but also with the origins of the universe. The force of silence is an immeasurable reality for science, yet its power can be seen in mathematics of quantum theory and is not limited in time to history or in space to the confines of this planet. That force has a subtle intelligence, some type of quantum mind.

After this dream, *The Quantum Mind and Healing* seemed the perfect title because, after all, that is how we experience mysterious body events and health issues that have until now been attributed to nature, God, the psyche, quantum processes (superposition of states, nonlocality, entanglement, etc.), or dark matter (the theoretical, invisible extra matter needed in the universe to explain its rate of change).

The relationship between physiology, medicine, physics, and psychology has been debated for years. The view in this book is that mathematical statements describing elementary particles, molecules, and human bodies are projections of dreaming experiences.

The Quantum Mind and Healing speaks to that part of you that is interested in understanding symptoms and working experientially with your own body symptoms and the somatic troubles of others. For the part of you suffering from such symptoms arising in connection to physical diseases, there are specific methods of approaching these symptoms and being enriched by them. For the scientist interested in integrating different fields, the viewpoint I present about science is simple: Human awareness is the first principle. How we notice things, that is, the nature of our perception and experience, is the basis of any observation or theory.

Writing this book brought me face to face with the most "realistic" part of myself, a part which sometimes ignores subjective experience. The conservative scientist within me thinks it is better to stick to one discipline in one lifetime. I agree. Yet because of my lifelong interest in working with body symptoms, something in me could not be tied down by the thoroughness required to pursue one discipline. I can only admit that to the best of my ability, I have tried to make this work as rational, reasonable, and understandable as possible.

My struggle reminds me of the words of Erwin Schrödinger, one of the parents of quantum mechanics. In the introduction to his little book, *What Is Life?* he says:

> A scientist is supposed to have a complete and thorough knowledge, at first hand, of some subjects and is usually expected not to write on any topic of which he is not a master. This is regarded as a matter of *noblesse oblige*. For the present purpose I beg to renounce the *noblesse*, if any, and to be freed of the enduing obligation. . . .
>
> It has become next to impossible for a single mind fully to command more than a small, specialized portion of [science]. . . . I can see no other escape from this dilemma (lest our true aim be lost for ever) than that some of us should

venture to embark on a synthesis of facts and theories—albeit with second-hand and incomplete knowledge of some of them—and at the risk of making fools of ourselves.

Dealing with symptoms leaves some of us no choice but to sew together what we know about psychology, medicine, physics, and spiritual traditions without having mastered all of them.

For these reasons, and to gain greater understanding of the body and of psychology, I have hesitated for more than twenty years, since writing *Dreambody*, to ground my understanding of how dreams connect with and influence body symptoms. In chapter 2 of *Dreambody*, published in 1982, I speak of how the dreambody has much in common with quantum theory. I said no more at that time, instead focusing mainly on the mythology of the dreambody. During the intervening twenty years, I have been satisfied with the results of psychological and somatic interventions with the dreaming body. I explored and extended basic ideas, making them applicable to working with individuals and groups in all states of consciousness. Today, my experiences, experiments, and practices with more than one hundred thousand people worldwide have brought me to the point of the present book: attempting to connect medicine and psychology with the physics of nonlocality.

Our bodies are localized where we are. On the other hand, the body is nonlocal, touched by relationships and groups, by immediate and stellar events. Not only do the human and natural environments touch us, but what happens within us changes our world. As you will learn as you move along with this book, such changes which are foretold in quantum theory now must become a part of a new quantum medicine, or nonlocal medicine. We cannot solve the problems in the body only by looking within the body. To solve some of our problems, we need to work with the whole world in the exact manner we experience it.

May this book bring the patient, the doctor, and the theoretician greater understanding and relief from physical pain.

Yachats, Oregon, 2002
www.aamindell.net

I
THE FORCE OF
SILENCE IN SYMPTOMS

1 The Force of Silence

If we don't dare to dream, we won't find anything. . . . Dreams are how the most exciting science happens.

—*Dan Goldin, chief of the U.S.
National Aeronautics Space Agency*[1]

Body symptoms are fierce battlegrounds full of intensity and trouble. If you deny your symptoms, you repress the battle and the symptoms spook you all night. On the other hand, if you focus only on their reality, you get depressed and fearful, especially if they are not immediately healed. *The Quantum Mind and Healing* presents principles which explain how and why working with your dreams and body sensations in a real and dreamlike manner changes your body experience.

Dear reader, my commitment to you is to make these princi-ples feel as plausible as possible to both your body and mind. My basic point is that your awareness interacts with the subatomic realm of your body. As an individual seeking resolutions to inner problems at the beginning of the third millennium, you must accomplish what our sciences have not yet accomplished. You must seek help not only from the growing domain of biomedicine, but also by exploring the deepest dreaming and quantum levels of your body. At these levels, you will meet what I call the force of silence, your body's intelligence and link to the universe.

To facilitate this exploration, I suggest various steps throughout the book to help you experience and understand your body and mind at this subtlest of all levels. Beyond supporting your personal journey, I also offer the suggestions of medical professionals and therapists, physicists and biologists, allopaths and alternative medical practitioners about how to unify existing paradigms. My direction is to integrate the ingenuity of today's sciences with yesterday's wisdom traditions. We shall be wandering through shamanism as well as quantum phenomena, psychology, and biochemistry, to outline new methods for understanding and working with symptoms.

Past and Present Work

In earlier books—*The Dreambody* and *Working with the Dreaming Body*—I demonstrated that dreams are mirrored in all kinds of body symptoms. In *Dreaming While Awake,* I suggested a shamanistic lifestyle based on lucid awareness 24 hours a day. In my recent *The Dreammaker's Apprentice,* I used Aboriginal Australian Dreamtime ideas and quantum theory to update what we therapists since Freud and Jung call "dreamwork."

Now, in *The Quantum Mind and Healing,* I unfold lessons of physics and psychology by reconsidering:

• Dreaming and the quantum dimension of symptoms,
• The origins of life and how awareness is an anti-aging factor,
• How quantum theory can be music therapy for symptoms,
• Why communities affect the body, and
• New, nontoxic lifestyles which promote wellness.

My ideas are the product of two factors: 40 years of experience working with people in all states of consciousness and with every conceivable body problem, and physics. For me, physics is a theory, a practical fact, and also a metaphor for our psychology. Math and physics are symbolic formulas describing deep altered states of consciousness as well as physical processes. New ideas arise in physics not only because of experimentation and theory, but because our consciousness is ready to discover new aspects of the universe within ourselves. In my earlier book, *Quantum Mind*, I have shown how everyone can experience physics. The math of physics is like the dream behind reality. Thus everyone can experience the immeasurable quantum wave fields in physics, because these virtual fields are maps of subtle body tendencies (as I will demonstrate below), as well as events in the real world.

While mainstream science focuses on measuring the effects of zero-point energy in the universe and debates whether or not subtle energy fluctuations gave rise to the origins of the universe, I will suggest a meditation on how the smallest inklings of awareness create our lives in terms of what I call the force of silence. In *Quantum Mind*, I discussed how these inklings are "tendencies" seen in quantum physics, psychology, and meditation. Self-reflecting patterns found in the math of physics—the basis of quantum theory—can be seen as metaphors for how the force of silence creates consciousness, reality, and all life's joys, problems, and symptoms.[2]

In this present book I show that these subtle, universal, and immeasurable tendencies create what we can sense in our bodies as the force of silence. Further, these tendencies are linked to the universe's self-reflecting ability as well as to our own. A conclusion about medicine follows from these insights: Training awareness, not curing illness, is the most basic task of medical practitioners. Body symptoms are not only problems to be solved. Chronic symptoms are *koans*—apparently unanswerable questions meant to increase our consciousness. Many such symptoms require dropping our everyday thinking and using awareness to perceive the force of silence in our bodies.

Today's mainstream biomedical viewpoint about the body reminds me of a city map. For example, on that map you will find a point representing your address, the location of your body. Most of us think of ourselves as located at some point on some map. The truth of this space and time viewpoint is obvious. However, this is not the whole truth.

In dreams, as in quantum theory, immeasurable yet experiential parts of you are not located only on a street corner, in a city, in a country on some continent or island on the planet Earth. Neither are you located only in this solar system or even in the Milky Way. Rather, you are located in consensus reality on that point of the map, *and* simultaneously in dreamland you are spread throughout the universe. For you to believe that your body is located solely at a particular spot on the planet may disturb your personal relationships and create symptoms as well.

The new medicine needs to discover and remember that whatever happens in this universe (or these parallel universes) influences our bodies, just as what we feel and think—how we experience things—touches the whole universe. We live in the universe, which is made up of real and virtual realities. Therefore the new medicine must be "local" and deal with the body in time and space, and "nonlocal" to deal with the way the world around us affects our bodies.

At the beginning of the twenty-first century, the everyday mind must object, telling us that quantum realities and subjective experiences are figments of our imagination and are not to be trusted. First, I want to relax this everyday mind by assuring it first that the present theory does include and affirm all that is known in present-day medicine and Newtonian physics and chemistry. I even suggest that the present work affirms quantum theory in a psychological way. Second, I suggest that ignoring subtle experiences symbolized in dreams and quantum theory may contribute to bodily *dis*-ease. In other words, you need experimentally verifiable medicine and physics as well as subjective experiences.

Exercise: Imaginary Time Experiment

How does knowing about the real and virtual quantum realities of the universe help my body problems in the here and now in a "down-to-Earth" fashion? *The Quantum Mind and Healing* answers this question with a theory and suggestions for ways to personally experience the theory.

Let's turn to experience first. The body experiment we are about to do encourages you to sense how the force of silence moves your body. After that, we discuss a theory about how this force was present at the origins of the universe in the realm of imaginary time.

Let me first add that since the force of silence, like all quantum-realm concepts in physics, is not directly measurable (only the effects can be tested in reality), you must use and depend on your own subjective experience and ability to sense things that are not "consented upon" by others. In what happens next, you may discover tendencies to think, imagine, and move in a specific direction, before you actually move in that direction.

Let's begin with your body awareness. To begin with, sit, stand, or lie in a position giving your body some freedom to move. If you are sitting, sit on the edge of your chair. If you are lying down, sit up a bit.

Now relax for a moment in your position. Take a couple of breaths. Don't rush. When you feel more at ease and a bit quieter, you are ready to go on.

While breathing freely and naturally, hold your body relatively still. Use your awareness to notice the kind of motion and direction your body might tend to move in if it were allowed. Don't move in that direction quite yet, just explore the tendency to move in a given way or direction. Give yourself time. The tendency will eventually show itself. Now, notice that tendency and its direction, even if this tendency seems unusual to you.

Once you notice it, allow that tendency to move your body slowly in that direction. Please take note of images which may arise. Take your time. What fantasies and images arise as you move?

Still moving slowly, follow your imagination about that movement until your inner images give you a sense of the movement's meaning. What could your tendencies, fantasies, and movements possibly mean for you? What meaning do they seem to have for you? Trust your intuition about the meaning. Focus your awareness on that possible meaning and make a note of it.

Finally, after noting this meaning, go back to the movement you were just making, and ask your body what body experiences, symptoms, or fears of symptoms it might produce to make you more aware of this tendency? What kind of symptom or fears of symptoms might express that tendency more dramatically so that you would have to look at it? Do you already have the beginnings of such symptoms, or are you afraid of such body states?

One of my clients who had been suffering from fears of death did this experiment at home by himself. He told me that his awareness made him realize that his body was "tending to relax, and his jaw wanted to drop." Then, after letting his jaw hang down, he had a sudden fantasy. His head fell off his body, leaving an image of his body breathing freely and totally open to the wind which could easily enter. He said: "The meaning was obvious: Drop my head, my inner programs, and open up." He reported that, to his surprise, his fears of death were resolved when he realized that his "head," or his rational mind, was trying to die!

This experiment may also have given you a sense of the kind of body tendencies that are present before movement occurs. Your sense of these tendencies is what I am calling the force of silence—a subtle force moving your body. Usually this subtle force makes itself known to you only when it appears in exaggerated forms such as fearful fantasies or body sensations.

The force of silence is both a subtle body sensation and the driving force behind your dreams, subtly trying to move you along a given path, giving life specific meanings. These meanings become clear only after looking back over your life or by getting in touch with that force in a given moment.

At the very least, not following the force of silence makes you uncomfortable, "dis-easy." Your body feels more at ease if you move with it, in the direction of its subtle force of silence.

Aspects of the Force of Silence

In the following chapters I show how this force appears not only in your body's subtle movement tendencies, but also within:

- Your chronic symptoms,
- Your long-term behavioral patterns, problems, and gifts,
- The moods and people that trouble you most, and
- Your relationship troubles or community problems.

The force of silence manifesting in tendencies is a kind of pull or push, coinciding in our awareness with the sensation of a kind of atmosphere, a mood, or field in which we are living. I call this atmosphere and its tendencies an "intentional field," though we are usually not aware of any intent behind the atmosphere or its subtle and easily ignored force of silence.[3]

I will show how focusing on such subtle experiences is a kind of *nonlocal* medicine, since these subtle tendencies may be connected not only to ourselves but to the whole world, indeed the whole universe.

Physics, Zen, and the Force of Silence

Let me begin to suggest a theory about how these experiences might connect within our universe. For the moment, let's begin with the assumption from physics that the basic pattern found in the subatomic realm for all matter—the quantum wave function— is one of the most basic patterns of our entire universe.

When Erwin Schrödinger, one of the grandparents of quantum theory, first discovered this wave pattern in the 1920s, he was certain it was "material." He called the mathematical waves of this pattern "matter waves." Today we know these waves are not material in the sense of measurable water waves. However, they are more fundamental than the apparent materiality of large-scale objects and bodies. This basic pattern is mathematically exact and predicts the probability that events will occur in everyday reality.

This wave function is typical of many quantum physics ideas that are very different from the Newtonian physics of events in everyday life. (See the sidebar below for more information about the wave function.)

Classical and Quantum Physics

Classical physics and medicine are closely connected with the cause-and-effect thinking of Isaac Newton, whose ideas come to us today from the late seventeenth century. What seems to be a ball in classical physics, or an object or body of any sort, is thought of as atoms and subatomic particles in quantum physics. In fact, the mathematics of quantum physics describes a world where causes and effects, not to mention the exact meaning of point and particle, are no longer certain.

Quantum physics is described by mathematical patterns that approximate what can be seen by an observer in everyday reality. The *position* and *velocity* of a particle, for example, cannot be measured precisely and simultaneously in everyday reality. Furthermore, there is no single way of understanding the mathematics of quantum physics.

In the February 2001 issue of *Scientific American,* in an article called "100 Years of Quantum Mysteries," award-winning black hole physicist John Wheeler and University of Pennsylvania physics professor Max Tegmark described what they called "the mysterious side of quantum physics": "Despite the early successes of the quantum idea, physicists still did not know what to make of its strange and seemingly ad hoc rules. There appeared to be no guiding principle. What was this 'wave function'? . . . This central puzzle of quantum mechanics remains a potent and controversial issue to this day."

In a statement that has made the Nobel Prize winner Richard Feynman almost notorious for his boldness, he suggested that if you think you understand quantum physics, you are kidding yourself. Feynman, possibly the greatest physicist since Einstein, said in his book *The Character of Physical Law,* "I think I can safely say that nobody understands quantum mechanics."

In any case, in quantum physics, a particle no longer fits our normal idea of a particle. Furthermore, there is no one interpretation of the wave function for particles—the mathematical pattern describing their behavior—because there is no certain way of measuring the equation. Most physicists believe, as does Werner Heisenberg, who discovered the uncertainty principle, that if you cannot measure the quantum world, you should not make firm statements about that world.

The patterns of quantum physics and its math are acceptable to scientists not because the basic equation, the so-called Schrödinger wave equation, can be measured and tested, but because it predicts statistically measurable results. Likewise in psychology, dreams, like mathematical patterns, cannot be exactly measured, and no one really knows exactly what they are. Nevertheless, dreams too predict the probable everyday behavior of dreamers. Even though a given interpretation may be debated, therapists and clinical psychologists the world over largely accept the idea of dreamwork.

Quantum theory is like the vision or dream an artist has before painting a picture. The artist may have a perfect image of the picture-to-be in a vision, but in the moment of painting the picture on canvas, unpredictable events occur. The final painting is unpredictable. Likewise, the quantum theory is a kind of vision of how the universe works. It gives general outlines, but not all the final details. In this book, I show how quantum theory is a vision not only of physical events but of psychological experience as well.

In thinking about the origins of the universe, cosmologist Stephen Hawking uses quantum wave patterns to understand the moment of creation. He suggests that at the beginning of time—when time was zero—"imaginary time" existed. Hawking uses this "dream" or vision because physics without quantum theory works well only back to the first 10^{-43} second after the universe began. Before that, non-quantum physics does not work. Hawking uses quantum waves as the "vision" or theory about the very first moment.

What happened at the beginning of the universe? Hawking suggests that an immeasurable "imaginary time" ruled the beginning of our universe, before there was "real" space, time, or matter.[4] His idea may not be so far out as it may seem. After all, you just experienced how subtle tendencies and patterns exist in your imagination and are present just before they produce real and measurable movements. At the beginnings of the universe, before there was physical reality as we know it, there may have been subtle, tiny, dreamlike experiences or tendencies in a kind of dreamlike or imaginary time.

As I have already suggested, it seems to me that quantum physics describes not only the material universe but the psychological as well. After working with thousands of people, I have found that all body movements and symptoms can be traced back to these tiniest, most subtle, "imaginary" experiences that precede their "real" everyday appearances. In a way, *symptoms* (and everything else in life) *begin in imaginary time, which can be felt as a subtle body signal—i.e., the force of silence.*

It was Werner Heisenberg, another parent of quantum theory, who first said that the quantum wave function behind physical reality represents an imaginary or immeasurable "tendency" towards reality. In other words, according to quantum theory and the views of some cosmologists, real events are described by, and arise from, immeasurable tendencies. A less complicated way of saying this is to speak as an Aboriginal person, saying that the world began in "Dreamtime." I call palpable effects of Dreamtime "the force of silence."

Dreamtime's force of silence is behind everything; it is one of the keys to understanding this world. The force of silence is an idea and an experience of the *earliest source* of events. To use this force—to learn to move with it and work with symptoms—you need only to learn to focus your awareness during stillness. Awareness is a core element in the sense of body wellness. Awareness may be the key to finding answers to many questions.

Zen and Dreaming

Awareness in reduced states of consciousness reminds me of how a friend of mine answered a most difficult question in life. This friend, Keido Fukushima, who lives in Kyoto, told me one of the stories behind his becoming a Zen master (and the head of the Rinzai sect of Zen Buddhism). While studying Zen, he was given a koan to answer by his teacher. When Keido heard the koan, at first he went deeply into himself. Following the unknown, his body began to dance in response to the koan!

His teacher was delighted with this "answer" and asked where the dance came from. While waiting for the answer, the teacher told my friend to leave the city they were in and live with the aboriginal group in Japan who danced in that manner. After years of living with that group, he became a Zen master. When his teacher died, Keido told me he did that dance for his teacher on his grave.

In a similar way, life is asking you many unanswerable questions. Your body is also trying to dance the answers. By learning to focus your awareness, you can use the unpredictable movements within you to resolve many seeming mysteries, including your body symptoms.

In a way, symptoms are koans asking you to let your body "dance," to use awareness and re-experience the deepest aspects of yourself. If your quantum wave is connected to the universe, your body's subtle movements are dancing in the rhythm of the universe as well.

About This Book

To explain these ideas more completely and give further suggestions for innerwork experiments, I have divided this book into parts focusing on work with individual symptoms and their connection to relationships, aging, and freedom in lifestyles.

In part 1, The Force of Silence in Symptoms, I show that medicine's central job is supporting awareness of the subtle forces of life. After studying quantum physics and psychology, as well as medical and spiritual approaches to the body, I talk about "Rainbow Medicine," which is a mixture of biomedicine, alternative traditions, and physics. Rainbow Medicine comes about through experiencing how life spontaneously arises, giving us the sense of wellness. Rainbow Medicine has many "colors." Many allopathic and alternative medicines are more monochromatic, that is, they have fewer levels and are more one color than a rainbow. "One-color" medicines include aspirin and vitamins, relaxation techniques and therapeutically derived resolutions to personal problems. "One-color medicine" is a crucial part of the greater picture which also includes dreaming.

Part 2, Nonlocal Medicine: The World in Symptoms, uses quantum physics and innerwork exercises to demonstrate just how your body is nonlocal—that is, everywhere you or someone else thinks you might be. Symptoms cannot always be healed by local medications directed to specific parts of your body, because the body problems you suffer from are, in a way, not solely your own—they also are found in relationships and community problems, in the past and even in the future.

Part 3, Aging: Chemistry, Buddhism, and Entropy, shows how the force of silence leads to new approaches toward aging, genetics, and ancestral bonds. I talk about how near-death or feared-death experiences can bring creativity to life. New views of life and death as simultaneous states appear now in psychology as well as physics.

Part 4, Quantum Demon Lifestyles: The Body Free of Time, introduces new methods of working with symptoms that involve multiple roles in relationship and shamanistic attitudes. The book concludes by reconsidering nonlocality and suggesting nontoxic lifestyles that integrate various levels of awareness. Here you find ideas summarizing *The Quantum Mind and Healing*.

In the appendices, which are geared for the scientifically interested reader, I tie together elementary concepts about waves, quantum physics, parallel worlds, and the quantum mind.

2 Rainbow Medicine

Something has to be added to the laws of physics and chemistry before the biological phenomena can be completely understood.

—*Werner Heisenberg*[1]

It is my personal opinion that in the science of the future reality will neither be "psychic" nor "physical" but somehow both and somehow neither.

—*Nobel Prize winner, Wolfgang Pauli*[2]

In this chapter, I suggest a unifying medical paradigm, "Rainbow Medicine," and show how its concepts are found not only in classical and alternative medicine, but in physics, spiritual experience, and in the study of altered states of consciousness as well. Rainbow Medicine is another name for multidimensional approaches in medicine.

Why do most of us feel bad for ourselves and others when we are ill? There are many possible reasons. One of the most troubling is that the part of us connected to consensus reality identifies illness as being *only* "real" or material (that is, as being very different from the world of dreams). Of course illness is real, and it disturbs your life. Serious illness may mean you can't work, which means losing money, and you suffer pain, perhaps feel a fair amount of fear, are unable to enjoy the people in your life, and so on. In short, without the force of silence and the dreaming layer of existence, everyday reality can be very one-sided and depressing.

Feeling bad for an ill person unwittingly identifies the sick person with only this everyday reality. Feeling bad for someone can be patronizing if you negate the unlimited power of dreaming imbedded in their symptoms and assume they are fundamentally powerless and dependent upon medical systems and fate.

Just about everyone is upset when faced with serious illness and perhaps even impending death. Nevertheless, in the world of dreams symptoms can reveal the most awesome messages from infinity. If you and I, as well as the practitioners of ordinary medicine, recognized both the real *and* the dreamland message of symptoms, those who fear negative diagnoses and attitudes would feel more appreciated and empowered and would be more likely to seek help.

The present standard medical attitude is partly responsible for discouraging many from getting the treatment they need (not to mention the cost, if you cannot afford insurance). In other words, if you are ill, you are ill *only* from the bio-medical perspective. From another, you are having big dreams in your body and (in a way) are lucky to receive dramatic messages from the force of silence.

Rainbow Medicine Is Multileveled

Just as the rainbow has many colors in it, the body—like all material objects—has various "colors" of reality in it. One "color" is that of "consensus reality," the tangible, physical aspects of biomedical reality to which we are all accustomed. In this reality, the "normal body" has a head, two arms, two legs, a heart, and so forth, and it is seen as an object located in time and space. However, like all material objects, the body has other "colors," other "frequencies."

The body has dreamlike dimensions that cannot be easily measured and located in time and space. We can measure body height, weight, and temperature, but we cannot directly measure or locate the body's quantum wave patterns or the subtle feeling that a given body may be having. Nevertheless, most people can feel subtle tendencies even before they manifest as recognizable patterns (as you may have experienced in the last chapter).

Rainbow Medicine includes the real time and real space of physical reality as well as dreamlike levels of the body's psychological reality. Rainbow Medicine includes components of classical medicine such as anatomy, diagnosis, medication, surgery, biophysics, etc., as well as alternative medical procedures involving subjective experience, dream patterns, and all levels of consciousness.

Rainbow Medicine deals with at least the following three levels of reality, each of which is linked to a particular form of awareness:

1. *Consensus reality:* observations of time, space, weight, and repeatable measurements.

2. *Dreamland:* experiences of fantasies, subjective feelings, dreams, and dreamlike figures.

3. *Essence:* perception of subtle tendencies and a lucid sense of the force of silence from which dreams arise.

Any medicine that deals with only one of these levels I call a "one-color medicine." Rainbow Medicine includes all levels of awareness.

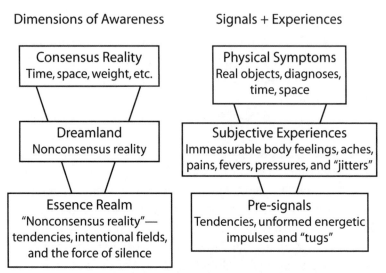

Figure 2-1. Rainbow Medicine and Its Three Levels of Awareness

Rainbow and One-Color Medicines

One-color medicine focuses mainly upon one or two dimensions. All cognitive therapeutic approaches, including allopathic (standard) medicine, deal mainly with the top area of figure 2-1, consensus reality. All medicines are needed; "alternative" and standard medicine are part of Rainbow Medicine. All the various areas are needed, and no one medicine is "better" than the other; they all belong to part of a more complete system.

In Rainbow Medicine, the different approaches to the body are linked to specific lifestyles (chapter 21 will deal with this in detail) and to ways of viewing and experiencing the universe. As I said, Rainbow Medicine, like the rainbow, is multileveled. To explain Rainbow Medicine thinking, let me ask a few questions. How do you explain why the seasons change? Do they just happen? Would you be satisfied with the answer the Earth's tilted axis allows for more direct sunlight in the summer and less in winter? Alternatively, are you more satisfied with poetic descriptions of why seasons change? Recall, for example, Simon and Garfunkel (or anyone else) singing "April, Come She Will."

Both the angle of the Earth's axis and the dreamlike feeling (e.g., "A love once new has now grown old") are needed to fully describe and explain the change of seasons. Both the consensus reality (CR) level and the dreamland level speak to different dimensions, different feelings about the seasons of time.

Likewise, we need to know about bacteria as well as dreams to understand life. Genes and bacteria explain a lot about what happens to us. However, dreams help explain the course of life in terms of imagery and meaning. Today's medicine is basically Newtonian, dealing mainly with consensus reality and largely ignoring subjective experience. Quantum mechanics is very different, though its most imaginary side remains "dubious" to most scientists. Quantum mechanics deals with invisible dimensions behind the ideas of matter. Both Newtonian biology and the real and invisible dimensions of quantum physics are part of Rainbow Medicine.

In nonrelativistic Newtonian physics—the old physics—matter is seen as a distinguishable entity in space, as a bunch of parts and particles. In quantum mechanics and the new physics, matter is seen as more ethereal; it is more like what scientists thought ether was—vague stuff that was supposed to fill the empty space of the universe. Today, with Einstein's relativity theory, we know that ether does not exist. Instead, we have phenomena like quantum vacuum fields. Matter itself is no longer just a hunk of something; it is an ethereal wave in an invisible space. In chapter 1, you got a hint about how these waves are not only abstract theories (or imaginary numbers in math) but also "tendencies" (as Heisenberg called them) or, more generally, "intentional fields" that can be felt.

The tendencies described in the mathematics of quantum physics are symbols that span the worlds of consensus reality and dreaming.[3] This math is a metaphor of abstract qualities as well as the forces of the dreaming, provoking us to certain directions in life.

Long before Western science was developed, Aboriginal healers in shamanic traditions everywhere experienced such directions as the guidance of some great spirit. I have personally met healers in Africa, Australia, the Americas, and India who actively use their awareness in the above three areas—consensus reality, dreamland, and the realm of essence. In a way, our ancestors have always known about and felt the quantum dimensions of the body without calling them such.

By itself, until now, Western science has had little to teach us about the mind or consciousness. In a way, Western psychology's insights into the mind began with Freud's conceptualization of the "subconscious." Today's neurosciences are exploring how and if consciousness can be reduced to the brain. The future seems clear to me; the next step for allopathic medicine will be to create a Rainbow Medicine that integrates physics, psychology, and biology with the wisdom from humankind's earliest religions.

The Rainbow Medicine "Doctor"

By redefining medicine, "doctors" will become awareness specialists. Imagine a future "rainbow doctor" who is able to work with the consensus-reality body and the dreaming body as well. She is a person you visit to help you with your health problems and dreaming.

Empowering your belief in yourself, she says, "My dear friend, your most difficult symptom is fascinating. You say you have aches and pressures in your body and are always fatigued. Well, we will explore these problems and listen to your body. Perhaps these symptoms are posing a question to you, a koan. Like a Zen master, your body has posed a question to you about life in the form of a symptom.

"How shall we find the answer to this koan? At present, the nature of this symptom is not completely understood by our standard medicine. We will investigate it in the allopathic tradition, but we need to get beyond what we know with our minds. This may be the moment you have been secretly waiting for; the challenge to contact your deepest nature. In a way, your symptoms may lead to some form of enlightenment."

If this is the first such rainbow doctor you have met, at this point you may be so shocked that you leave her office. But then, as times and cultures change and Rainbow Medicine practice becomes more common, you might feel relieved. You no longer need to choose between sciences and mystical traditions, between allopathic or alternative medicine, since aspects of all paradigms will be considered in your doctor's—awareness specialist's—office. The concepts of health and the pathology of illness are still in this office, but they have become one-color medicine concepts and relate to the everyday you in consensus reality who wants to live to a ripe old age. In Rainbow Medicine, you are neither ill nor well, young nor old, but simply on a path, of whose intent you are not yet conscious.

Perhaps your doctor will say next that "Your symptoms of fatigue and persistent aches and chest pressure are the beginnings of a dance. Let your body dance and express whatever is in your chest creating that pressure."

You insist that you don't dance well, and especially not in front of anyone. However, she tells you to relax and shows you what she means by letting her hands express something that looks to you like a puppet creating pressure by pushing something away. She suggests following the slightest impulses in your body. Before you know it, your body has stood you on your feet and you are dancing. You feel like and become a great giant banging on the confining walls of his dwelling, wanting to get out. "Let me out, let me out!" Your doctor asks, "Why?" and you answer, without knowing why, "Let me out! I am too big to be cooped up in this chest! I am not tired, I am exploding with energy, and I've got a big job to do!"

What a surprise. Before your dance, you thought you were fatigued. Now you feel energized. A few minutes later you discover what your job is: You want to change something specific in yourself or others around you, or perhaps the "giant" wants to do something you thought was delusional, like changing your city.

In any case, you go home feeling better and take up the challenge. You no longer need some form of medication to support or retard that giant. Better yet, you feel enriched by the awareness those symptoms brought you, and you feel better, with or without your allopathic medicine—and even if the symptoms reappear.

Classical and Rainbow Medicine

Today's medicine classifies diseases as either infectious or noninfectious. Microorganisms like bacteria and viruses are seen as upsetting the body and creating infectious diseases. Noninfectious diseases are considered due to one or more causes. If the causes are unknown—as is the case, for example, with some cancers and obesity—it is believed that the causes will be found. Age, genetics, culture, economics, geography, and climate are all recognized as playing important roles in disease.

Some one hundred years ago, the main causes of death were smallpox, tuberculosis, and cholera. Now in the more technically developed countries today, degenerative diseases such as heart problems and neoplastic disorders dominate morbidity statistics. Causal factors creating disease are being discovered and uprooted, allowing us to face new problems of aging and the psychological and spiritual elements associated with disease.

Alternative medical procedures such as Chinese medicine, homeopathy, chiropractic medicine, and others have been working with the noncausal and psychological or spiritual factors connected with disease for centuries. Theories of "energy" are now competing with theories of "information" as paradigms for explaining how the body's components may communicate with one another along a sort of continuum, which makes the real body more of a blur than a fixed object.

Classical medicine has gained much from Newtonian physics, which seeks to understand the linear and local causes behind events (those which are within reach of our physical senses). There are causes that do have effects in the everyday world. If you push a ball on a flat surface, the ball rolls. Likewise, your body changes if it is physically pushed by someone or by some material or chemical. The cause-and-effect paradigm that characterizes much of medicine and classical physics has enabled us to double the length of human life (in the more technically developed countries) from what it was 120 years ago.

In the Rainbow Medicine approach, the origin of diseases may lie not only in simple or even multiple consensus-reality causes, such as bacteria, but in the force of silence. In this way, a Rainbow Medicine approach explains what causal paradigms cannot: why some diseases disappear and others continue on their lethal course; why our bodies sometimes recuperate spontaneously and at other times do not; why medications work with you in one state of mind but not in another.

My point is that Rainbow Medicine includes allopathic ideas of disease and illness, fatigue and pressure, health and material causation *alongside* shamanistic ideas—spirit in symptoms, "subtle energy" concepts such as "vital flow," "chi," "prana," "life force," and all the other terms healers across the centuries have used to describe body experience. Rainbow Medicine affirms modern science *and* develops the connections between homeopathy, anthroposophical medicine, and osteopathic and chiropractic traditions that appreciate the multidimensionality of individual experience. It is not a matter of "this but not that"; it is a principle of "this *and* that."

Rainbow Medicine and Spiritual Experience

When I first became interested in the healing potential of quantum tendencies, I thought to myself, "If these tendencies are so essential to feeling well, they must be found not only in the fundamental concepts of modern science but in religion and spiritual traditions as well."

For example, in Taoism you find the multileveled concepts characteristic of Rainbow Medicine approaches to life. The force of silence is very similar to the Tao concept in Lao Tse's ancient *Tao Te Ching,* namely, the mysterious "Tao that cannot be said." According to the Sinologist Harold Roth, earliest Chinese ideas about the Tao (predating the *Tao Te Ching*) define it as "the way," "meaning," as well as "vital essence."[4] According to Roth, this idea of the Tao "is the basis of health, vitality and psychological well being." The Tao is the "one," the "unhewn," the "simple," a "guiding force through our whole lives," which unfolds into the world of the ten thousand things.

Here indeed are Rainbow Medicine concepts—"vital essence," "the basis of health," and "a guiding force through life." Roth quotes an early description of the Tao, which sounds close to a description of how quantum waves not only describe but bring elementary particles and the whole universe to life:

The vital essence of all things,
It is this which brings them to life.
It generates the five grains below
And becomes the constellated stars above.
When flowing in the heavens and the Earth
They call it the numinous.
When stored in the chest of human beings,
They call it the sages.[5]

The "sages," the Tao in one's chest, is what I have called the force of silence. In the previous example, the Tao was the dance waiting to be realized. In the foregoing quote, this inner wisdom in our bodies is the same as that in the stars.

Altered States and Rainbow Medicine

Later, Chuang Tsu interpreted the "Tao that cannot be said" as the "primal force." This force is the palpable experience of movement tendencies that produce a sense of flow and easy movement or wellness. Gaining access to these tendencies produces an altered state of everyday consciousness. In the relaxed, open-minded state that is accompanied by lucid awareness, you approximate a central experience found in many spiritual traditions, an experience of oneness where things get done without you "doing" them.

Empty openness is called *Mu-shin* in Zen Buddhism and *Rigpa* in Tibetan Buddhism. Tibetan Buddhist Lama Sogyal Rinpoche speaks of a pre-dreaming or Rigpa state as the "essential, unaltered mind, a sort of intelligence which lies behind all things, and which can be experienced by relaxing, releasing your mind and bringing it home." In the Rigpa state, the mind's "innermost essence, which is absolutely and always untouched by change or death . . . could be said to be the knowledge of knowledge itself."[6]

Rigpa is the awareness of an experience of the "essence" from which all things arise and are created. In the Rigpa state, the sentient essence of events—the "intelligence of the universe"—

appears. One senses the nonlocal, all-present aspect of any so-called "everyday" event. In this state, a flower is not just a flower; instead, as the Aboriginal Australians might say, you discover "flower dreaming," its timeless power.

Just as a particle, according to quantum physics, can be anywhere at any time before it is observed, in the state of Mu-shin or Rigpa, according to Zen and Tibetan Buddhism, you can sense a subtle nonlocal "pre-face" to every real event. You connect to events in your dreaming or in your heart before they have manifested in everyday reality.

Rainbow Medicine and Zen As Creativity

Keido Fukushima once showed a class of mine this state of consciousness when he meditated for a while before painting—that is, doing his calligraphy. He sat in the middle of the room, meditating, with his brush and paper in front of him. Then, when he was in the "right" state, he picked up the brush, and in a minute the painting was done. In this state, he showed how the painter can let these subtle tendencies guide his brush.

There are many names, with slight variations in meaning, for this Rainbow Medicine state. To mention just a few, there is the state of oneness experienced as Brahman in Hinduism, the Great Spirit of the Native American beliefs, the God of Judeo-Christian and Muslim traditions.

Fukushima Roshi explains the Mu-shin state as "creative mind," though the more usual English translations are "no-mind," "emptiness," or "nothingness." "Creative mind" makes a lot of psychological sense to me, because when your mind is tuned in to the force of silence, when you sense tendencies, you are at once empty and in a highly attentive and creative state.

In this state, the thoughts, perceptions, and feelings of your everyday self no longer dominate your awareness, and you become open to the subtle and unpredictable fluctuations (in your body and all of the natural world). Altered "spiritual" states open one to a kind of primordial creativity where unpredictable fantasies and movements can occur.

Rainbow Medicine in Physics

Acclaimed physicist David Bohm added a spiritual or psychological dimension to quantum mechanics when he re-conceived quantum waves in terms of what he called "pilot waves," which he imagined somehow informed or guided material objects. He said that the wave function (or what I have been referring to as the force of silence) was a kind of guiding force that informed particles about where to go, just as a radar wave guides ships at sea. Though other physicists (particularly Werner Heisenberg) warned scientists that they should eschew any definitive conceptualizations about the wave function because it was immeasurable,[7] Bohm (and many other physicists) dared to think beyond the measurements of consensus reality.

Rainbow Medicine is found not only in spiritual experiences and alternative medical ideas, but also in the theories of physics. Rainbow Medicine is multidimensional; it includes subtle guiding waves, awareness of the Tao, Mu-shin, Rigpa, and similar immeasurable states, as well as an appreciation of concrete Newtonian physics and body chemistry.

The force of silence is a guiding creative intelligence that can be found in special states of consciousness and used to discover our creative edges. From this state of silence, tendencies first appear subliminally, then as pre-signals, and finally as tiny "flirts" catching your attention. In ordinary, everyday awareness, we tend to ignore these flickering pre-feelings and tiny body sensations because they are subtle, irrational, or short-lived. When we are in open states of lucid attention, however, these impulses are easily perceived.

Exercise: Flirts As Rainbow Medicine

Try the following experiment. Keep a pencil and piece of paper at hand.

Open your mind. For a few minutes, close your eyes, relax, and focus on how you are breathing. Don't rush forward, but take your time until you reach a kind of "zero state" of stillness.

Experience the flirt. Now, still lucid and open-minded, slowly open your eyes—or rather, let your eyelids open very slowly on their own. Gaze about the space you are in. Let your unconscious mind choose the object or experience that flickers in your gazing attention and hold that particular flicker or flirt. It may be subtle, and with your eyes in a foggy state, even vague. You may find yourself ignoring it at first. Use your awareness and hold that flirt in your mind's eye.

Focus on whatever caught your attention. Reflect upon the object or event for a moment or two. What is it? What does it remind you of? What does it feel like or look like?

Let the force of your dreaming unfold. Remain focused on that object or event and notice what is happening to it (or within it), until you almost know why you are "dreaming" about this flirt.

Pick up your pencil and let your hand quickly sketch something. To help understand your dreaming, make a spontaneous motion with your hand or your pencil on paper to express the energy of your dreaming.

Guess about the possible meaning of your dreaming. What is behind those images and experiences? What is significant for you in that dreaming in this moment? Make a note about this on the paper.

Feel the force of silence. When you are ready, ask yourself where the same pattern that appeared in that flirt has appeared in your recent inner or outer life experiences. Feel the tendency, the pilot wave, the force of silence that appeared to you in that flirt, and imagine a body symptom that this creativity might be connected to or resolve. Let that force move you in some way.

In special states of awareness, the force of silence appears as a creative urge that may be connected to a symptom. Connecting to the force of silence is a kind of medicine for you. If you are not careful, you can easily marginalize the subtle impulses because they seem so flickering at first, so evanescent or insignificant to you. Yet learning to focus on these states and fields, together with other methods of caring for yourself, is Rainbow Medicine.

3 Nanoflirts and Body Wisdom

In a classic talk[1] ushering in the era of nanoscience, Richard Feynman spoke at the annual meeting of the American Physical Society on December 29, 1959, saying: "The principles of physics . . . do not speak against the possibility of maneuvering things atom by atom. . . . In practice, it has not been done because we are too big. . . . I am not afraid to consider the final question as to whether, ultimately—in the great future—we can arrange the atoms the way we want."

In the previous chapter, flickerings, tiny perceptions, sensations, or flirts were found to carry a great deal of intelligence. These tiny flirt-like perceptions are a kind of "nano-awareness"— that is, awareness of the tiniest, most subtle experiences.

My Relative's Flirts

The following story pops into my mind about flirts. One day when I got bored talking to one of my relatives at a family gathering, I told him the kind of work I do and asked him to try out an exercise I had in one of my books. While we both sat on the couch, I suggested that he relax and just focus on his breathing. After a minute, I suggested that he scan his body and tell me about anything, even the tiniest thing that caught his attention. After a short pause he said, he did not understand why, but there was something like "dryness" in his throat. "It's too small to be a bother, but that is what you asked for," he assured me.

I suggested he focus on this dryness, since it had flirted with his attention. I told him I understood that he was not the kind of person who paid much attention to these silly fantasies, but he should try to do so now. I said something like, "Focus on that tiny little sensation that just appeared when you gave attention to your body. Re-experience it, even amplify it until you can easily imagine it."

He closed his eyes, wrinkled up his forehead as if he were thinking seriously about something, and then smiled and opened his eyes. With great excitement, he told me that as he focused on the dryness, he saw himself in a vast dry area: "It was a desert . . . no—it was a Native American sitting on the floor of a vast desert. Isn't that a strange fantasy?"

Barely hiding my own excitement, I asked him what the figure in the desert was doing. My relative said, "He was . . . well . . . kind of listening to what he imagines to be the voices of his ancestors speaking to him . . . telling him to let go of all his relationship troubles and not feel responsible for everyone!" At this point he was beside himself. He was shocked and laughed, telling me that he always felt overly responsible for everyone around him. He said, "The voice of that Native American ancestor in that dry desert must have been talking to me!"

I said, "What's wrong in feeling responsible?" He answered, "Something must be wrong with that. Every time I take care of someone, I have fits of coughing—how is this connected to the sense of dryness?" I suggested he knew the answer to this question himself. After a moment he said, "Ah-ha! I should not *feel* responsible but *be* more responsible to the 'ancestors.'"

This story illustrates several points:

29

- Tiny sensations or flirts are the beginnings of creativity and fantasy, stories and dreams. (Dryness in the throat led to an image of "a Native American sitting on the floor of a vast desert.")

- Flirts are the basis of symptoms. (The dryness was connected to the coughing fits.)

- Flirts are the core or essence of symptoms, and at the same time, their medicine. (The sensation of the dry throat offered the recipe for relieving his cough: being with the "ancestors" instead of being a caretaker.)

- Symptoms are their own medicine.

Nano-awareness and Medicine

Neither physics nor psychology has made enough out of these tiny, nano-like events until now. In a way, the minuscule flirts are to psychology what the movements of electrons and atoms are to physics. We could say that flirts are to psychology what nano-events are to physics.

Richard Feynman, the father of nanoscience, suggested that the reason we have not tried to do such things is because we are "so big." In the same way, by focusing mainly upon the verbal experiences and stories of people, psychology has focused mainly on events in nighttime dreams and consensus reality and has neglected individual and apparently meaningless subtle signals until they become so large that they can be "talked about."

Let me suggest here (and later discuss more concretely with the idea of the quantum state crossover in chapter 9) that the "psychology of flirts" is the subjective experience of nano-body events. Science and psychology ignored this area until now because mainstream thinking and living is oriented toward consensus reality (CR). This CR reality is, essentially, a bull in the china shop of nano-events. By focusing only on repeatable consensual kinds of events, our minds become clumsy and easily

Nanoscience

The term nano- is used as a prefix in science, to mean the one-billionth part of a unit, 10^{-9} degree, or .000000001. For instance, a nanometer is 10^{-9} meters, or .000000001 meters. This is the approximate size of an atom. A nanosecond is 10^{-9} seconds.

Nanoscience and technology can count the movement of a few electrons or move individual atoms around on the surface of different materials by using atomic force microscopes and scanners. Today, this new field is remodeling the forms of chemistry and medicine that are based on changing groups of molecules instead of working with individual atoms within a structure, such as bone.[2] Quantum physics gave rise to nanoscience and uses micro-scopes and scanners to explore parts of tissues and materials only a few atoms wide.

Medical science deals mainly with molecules and cells. However, nanomedicine will change the very positions of atoms. As nanomedicine grows, many drugs and medicines that mainly reorganize molecules and cells will no longer be necessary. I agree with Robert Freitas when he says in the foreword of the first volume of his book on nanomedicine, "The coming ability to carry out targeted medical procedures at the molecular level will bring unprecedented power to the practice of medicine. Within a few short decades, we can expect a major revolution in how the human body is healed."[3]

bypass the tiniest subtle, flirt-like experiences that precede dreamland and everyday reality.

Exercise: Exploring Nano-awareness and Body Wisdom

Immense changes can occur by our honoring the tiniest perceptions. We already know from the "Imaginary Time" exercise at the end of chapter 1 that the force of silence appears in the slightest movement tendencies. The "Flirts As Rainbow Medicine" experiment at the end of chapter 2 focused on how the force of silence organizes visual flirts. The following exercise will explore flickering, nano-like proprioceptive body sensations which appear to you in a more or less ordinary state of consciousness.

> *Take a moment, feel your body, and get in touch with your breath.* Now notice whatever little tiny body sensation is "asking" to be noticed. Notice "flickering," flirt-like, or sudden body sensations.
>
> *Now focus your whole awareness on that little thing.* Track the sensations, letting them unfold as they will. Feel them, see them, or hear them. Do not stop how they are unfolding with your conscious doubts or explanations.
>
> *Experiment with your nano-awareness.* Let those sensations unfold in a fanciful manner, until they have some meaning for you.

Was what you experienced somehow connected to body symptoms you have now (or have had in the past)? How is the flirt that you noticed possibly a core experience of that symptom? In what way could this core experience or essence enrich your life?

Your nano-body experiences can be doors to new spaces and states of consciousness. Symptoms are connected to your psychology and to your most special "powers." A symptom's flirts can be a "medicine"—in the greatest sense of the word—for life as a whole.

Quantum Waves and Consciousness

I know, from many years of practicing therapy as a process worker, working with people in all states of consciousness, that noticing and reflecting on nano-like experiences creates expanded consciousness. There is great wisdom embedded in body sensations and symptoms. However, physics and medicine are still not certain about what awareness means or what consciousness is.

I think of awareness in terms of the almost automatic and mostly involuntary perception of elementary sensations. If we develop awareness, we can become almost conscious in the world

Consciousness in Physics

John von Neumann was perhaps best known for his development of the EDVAC computer that is basic to computers of today. However, he was also one of the first great mathematicians of quantum physics. He stated clearly in the 1930s that consciousness entered the equations of physics—though he did not know where that location might be. Others, like the Nobel prize-winning physicist Eugene Wigner, said that consciousness somehow created reality. Today, other physicists agree.

The "Science of Consciousness" conferences at the University of Arizona are representative of a new movement in science, as are the *Journal of Consciousness Studies* (published by Imprint Academic in the UK), the *Journal of Frontier Sciences* (published by Temple University in Philadelphia), and many other individuals and institutions.

In *Shadows of the Mind* (1994), leading cosmologist Roger Penrose states: "A scientific worldview which does not profoundly come to terms with the problem of conscious minds can have no serious pretensions of completeness. Consciousness is part of our universe, so any *physical theory* which makes no proper place for it falls fundamentally short of providing a genuine description of the world." I would maintain that there is, as yet, no physical, biological, or computational theory that comes very close to explaining consciousness.

If you are interested in pursuing the study of consciousness in physics, you might begin with Neils Bohr's *Atomic Physics and Human Knowledge* (1958). The most basic thinking can be found in Werner Heisenberg's *The Physicist's Conception of Nature* (1958). Next, see Stuart Hameroff and Roger Penrose's 1996 article "Orchestrated Reduction of Quantum Coherence in Brain Microtubules: A Model for Consciousness." A grand overview is given by Roger Penrose in *The Emperor's New Mind* (1989) and *Shadows of the Mind* (1989).

of dreaming. In that moment we are "lucid"—as in lucid dreaming. I reserve the term "consciousness" for more everyday voluntary activities such as the ability to speak about experience. Consciousness is based upon awareness.

Participants in Consciousness

Imagine a system looking at itself, or better yet, you looking at yourself, or best of all, two objects, like you and your teacup, about to "look at" each other. The solid arrow in the following diagram represents observation. The dashed arrows below you and the cup represent the flirt that occurs between objects, such as you and the cup, before they realize they are observing one another.

Whereas the process represented by the thick black arrow can be tracked by a video camera as a signal exchange between you and your cup, you cannot track the flirts. You can only feel them "tapping you on the shoulder," making you quickly look at the cup. The dashed lines represent the flirt-ing—the subtle, nonconsensual interactions—between objects in everyday life once an observation has been consciously created, so you can say, "I look at my teacup."

The flirting phenomenon is implied in the mathematics of physics. According to Seattle physicist John Cramer, of the University of Washington, the two dashed lines above might be understood as waves in an imaginary realm. He suggested understanding what happens during the process of observation in terms of "reflecting offer and echo waves" that pass between observer and observed, or between the observer and herself.[4] Remember, you cannot measure these imaginary waves in everyday reality. They are

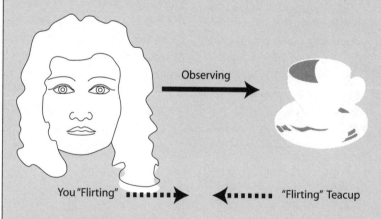

You "Flirting" ■■■■■■■▶   ◀■■■■■■■ "Flirting" Teacup

Observing

Figure 3-1. Observation

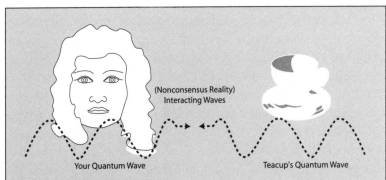

Figure 3-2. Interacting Waves

mathematical concepts that we refer to as waves because they are wave-like in an imaginary number realm. These waves may be understood as going both forward and backward in time.

Sound like science fiction? Yes. Now in psychology, the idea of science "fiction" no longer exists. As in the new physics, anything that can *possibly* be real—that is, anything that can be imagined—*is* real in another dimension. Flirts exist in nonconsensus reality which means that there is not likely to be a consensus on their existence among people living in large cities in the twenty-first century. You cannot catch flirts with a video camera.

In any case, along with Cramer, we can picture flirts (in nonconsensus reality) as the two quantum waves.

In the math of physics, these waves have equal strength and frequency but flow in opposite directions. According to Cramer, their interaction is something like the interaction between telecommunications machines, a sort of "handshake" which must occur before communication occurs. These two waves are then forgotten, just as the buzzes and beeps that precede faxes and e-mail are forgotten once you are finally online.

In the mathematics behind the process of observation in physics, these two waves multiply, creating a probability that something will be where we usually expect it to be, such as a particle being in a certain position at a certain time. Before observation, these immeasurable quantum waves are nonlocal, spread out all over the universe; after observation, they become the probability descriptions of real things localized in time and space.

Although today's physicists do not yet know and cannot explain why these waves must reflect mathematically to produce probabilities of location in reality, I suggested a reason.

Reflecting quantum waves mirror how we reflect tiny flirts when they catch our attention. Only after a flirt has been reflected by us, that is, has caught our attention, do we consider observing the object "producing" the flirt. A tree flirts with our attention, and we unwittingly attend to it with a reflecting flirt. The result of this reflection is what we call an observation in everyday life. However, once something is observed, we forget the subtle flirts behind the observation. Learning to focus upon flirt-like experiences, honoring and reflecting upon them, allows the wisdom inherent in them to emerge. This is a central theory of how nano-awareness, body wisdom, and consciousness are all connected.

In brief, quantum physics is based upon a self-reflecting tendency in the universe. The universe reflects upon itself; quantum waves, tendencies, or the force of silence reflect upon themselves, creating the everyday world. You can notice this happening in your psychology. You normally feel that you decide to notice things. However, through introspection or meditation training, you can discover that things first "tap you on the shoulder." They flirt with you *just before* you turn and look at them. Aboriginal peoples speak about the self-reflection of nature in terms of objects having animistic "powers" that make us look at them. In figures 3-1 and 3-2, I illustrate how things "tap us on the shoulder" before, or at the same time, we turn to look at them.[5]

Many physicists have suspected that intelligence, imagination, and great power exist somewhere in the universe. Einstein said, "I want to know God's thoughts . . . the rest are details." David Bohm formulated his belief in a great power when he said, in 1959, "The substructure of matter very probably contains energies that are as far beyond nuclear energies as known nuclear energies are beyond chemical energies. . . . [Zero-point] energy provides a constant background which is not available at our level under present conditions. But as conditions of our universe change, a part of it might be made available at our level."[6]

These thoughts about the power of zero-point energies and related quantum fluctuations sound like what has always been known by our Aboriginal relatives: "You listen, white man. Something is there; we do not know what; something like engine, like power, plenty of power; it does hard-work; it pushes."[7]

Waves, Snakes, and Medicine

The power of the universe is found not only in the quantum waves of physics but in the serpentine waves of mythology as well. The fundamental power of two interconnecting waves has been a symbol of medicine for centuries.

In figure 3-3, there are two snakes curled up in opposite directions on a staff. This symbol, called the "caduceus," is a wand or staff with two serpents entwined around it, surmounted by two wings. This staff is the symbol of the medical profession and of the medical branches of the U.S. Army and Navy.

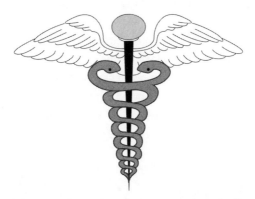

Figure 3-3. The Caduceus, Representing Healing

Hermes, messenger of the gods in Greek mythology, carried this staff and with it conducted the souls of the dead to the underworld and exercised magical powers over human sleep and dream times. In other words, the caduceus was the symbol of the power to move backward and forward—between life and death, wakefulness and dreams, consensus reality and dreamland. Today, the

The Medical Staff

According to *Taber's Cyclopedic Medical Dictionary*, the symbol of two intertwined snakes appeared early in Babylonia around 4,000 years before Christ and represented fertility, wisdom, and healing. According to Marie Louise von Franz in her *Time: Rhythm and Repose*, because the snake spends time beneath the surface of the earth but can also be rejuvenated through the shedding of its skin, it was associated in Greece with the human soul essence and was used to represent the soul after death.

The idea of the snake as the source of life is found in Egyptian mythology, where the snake is often pictured coiled around the tree of life, as the life essence. Later, Greek heralds and ambassadors carried this staff because of the supposed inviolability of the symbol; its carriers were protected from attack. Later, the caduceus became a Roman symbol for truce, neutrality, and noncombatant status.

caduceus is also used as a symbol of commerce, postal service, and ambassadorial positions.

This medical (and communication or postal service) symbol of the caduceus image of two snakes facing one another reminds me of the (conjugated[8]) quantum waves in physics (the basis for communication and perception) and of flirts, the basic "substance" of healing in Rainbow Medicine. At the quantum level, there is a symmetry in time, meaning that events may go either backwards

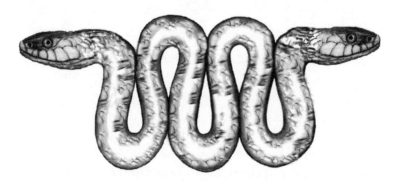

Figure 3-4. The Forward and Backward Nature of Time

or forwards in time. This corresponds to confusion about the subtle nature of relationship signals; we can often not tell exactly who did what first!

In any case, the double nature of the snake or the symmetrical quality of time appears in the New World symbolized by one snake with two heads, one representing life and the other death. Figure 3-4 is an artist's rendering of a Mexican double-headed serpent from around the thirteenth to fourteenth centuries (see von Franz's *Time: Rhythm and Repose*, figure 9, for more).

Flirts and Kundalini

The phenomenon of flirts seems to have been intuited long ago by our ancestors. In China, such waves were connected to the dragon lines of the Tao and to the subtle *chi* energies.

In India, this energy is *sat* (actually *sat-chi-ananda*) or *kundalini* serpent energy. Figure 3-5 indicates the kundalini energy

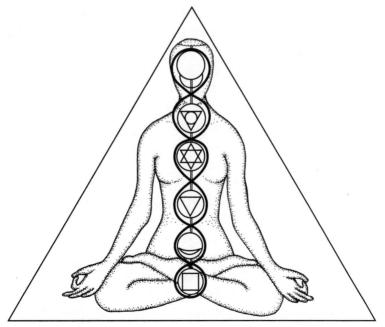

Figure 3-5. Kundalini Serpent Energy

awakening in a practitioner, rising through the various body centers or *chakras*, finally leaving the head to join the individual with the infinite being, the *Atman*.

In the practice of tantric yoga, meditation is used as a way to get in touch with or awaken this serpent energy and then to connect with the nonlocal personality, the experience of being everything, everywhere.

It seems to me as if the experience of kundalini energy flowing up the spine is an individual (nonconsensual) version of the physicists' image of the wave function and its fluctuating or flirt-like energy and tendencies. In a private meeting in the 1960s with my psychology teacher, Jungian analyst M. L. von Franz, and the eminent physicist from the Central European Research Agency in Switzerland, Carl F. von Weizsaecker, I was amazed to observe that Weizsaecker was fascinated by the connections between the fields of psychology and physics. I was *not* surprised recently to discover the following quote from Weizsaecker wherein he calls the Indian (or Hindu) kundalini energy of *prana*[9] a subtle "moving potency" and compares it with the wave function.[10] I am certain this analogy must have occurred not only to Weizsaecker, but to many other physicists as well. From his *What Is Life,* I know how important Indian philosophy and Vedanta were to Erwin Schrödinger (the discoverer of the wave equation).

For centuries, our ancestors worldwide sensed some form of wavy or serpentine energy as the base of our subtle physiology. Today, with encouragement to focus on immeasurable experience, we can feel subtle sensations, impulses, pulses, or pulsatile vibrations—*"something like engine, like power"* (in Aboriginal terms)—which seem to us to exist beneath the surface of consciousness in the body (just as the snake can be on the surface or beneath the earth).

To some of us, these vibrations may seem to be no more than barely perceptible wiggles or spasms, palpitations or electrical jitters. However, to others these subtle sensations have mythic significance. For example, Siddha yogi meditation practitioners such as the late Swami Muktananda experienced these sensations in terms of the subtle power of the goddess Shakti.

Siddha Yoga

The Siddha yogi Swami Muktananda, whom I respect as one of my teachers, referred to kundalini as Shakti, thereby equating kundalini energy with the female generative principle in Hindu mythology. In Muktananda's words (in his *Play of Consciousness,* page 18): "Shakti ... is the sounds, vibration of the Absolute, which manifested the universe. She brings language ... into existence ... has the power to create this universe. . . . She is the willpower of God. . . . She is Kundalini ... always playing ... she ... illuminates herself and makes herself known."

Kundalini-Shakti is the goddess image of flirts. She is a self-illuminating energy—the sound, the power, the engine, creating the real world. She is an image of "serpent power," a mythic counterpart to creation in imaginary time, to what cosmologists like Stephen Hawking refer to as the imaginary time dimension of quantum waves present at the beginning of the universe.

According to Muktananda: "Just as a seed contains a whole tree in potential form, Kundalini contains all the different forms of yoga, and when She is awakened through the grace of the Guru, She makes all yogas take place within you spontaneously. This is enlightenment."

Muktananda experienced what I call the force of silence as Shakti, the origin of spontaneous motions and consciousness. In the first chapter, I spoke of this energy in terms of tendencies and the intentional fields we feel in our bodies before movement occurs. When these subterranean impulses and pulses are followed, the subtlest movements seem to unfold into new worlds.

The analogies between mythology and physics are fascinating. We must notice that Kundalini-Shakti is pictured as two equal and opposite waves creating healing and consciousness, just as the wave function is pictured as two equal and opposite waves creating reality. Furthermore, Shakti is the "seed" or essence of the world, just as cosmologists consider the wave function to be the beginning of the universe.

Parallels between your flickering subtle body sensations (flirts), the dreamland origins of reality, quantum waves, and the

Kundalini–Shakti energy point to several aspects of these barely liminal sensations.

1. Your flickering body sensations are first stages of conscious experience.

2. These early stages are symbolized by serpent-like symbols and the mathematics of waves.

3. The serpent or wave essence self-reflects.

4. Through self-reflecting, She creates consensus reality based upon subatomic, subliminal body wisdom.

Kundalini, *chi,* caduceus symbology, serpent power, tendencies, intentional fields, quantum waves—all are concepts and images of everyone's almost unimaginable spontaneity and creativity. In those moments when you connect with the subtle force of silence, you may sense that former health fears were nanosignals, gateways to a new kind of wisdom.

4 Symptom Hyperspaces

... we must begin our analysis with an infinite
number of all possible universes, coexisting with
one another.

—*Physicist Michio Kaku*[1]

Two centuries ago, many people might have associated
Rainbow Medicine with witchcraft or the sacrilegious nature of
"modern science." Today Rainbow Medicine is simply multidimensional medicine. Whereas one-color medicine focuses mainly on
one or two dimensions of awareness, Rainbow Medicine includes
all awareness levels.

Though times are changing quickly in the direction of a larger
medicine, today mainstream medical attitudes generally focus on
the physical, spatial, and temporal aspects of what is characterized as "illness." Psychological approaches usually avoid the
physical body and focus on behavioral or dreamlike (transpersonal
and spiritual) experiences. One-color medicine and one-color
psychology focus on one, or at most two dimensions or "spaces"
of awareness.

In this chapter, I discuss how multidimensional awareness is connected to the experience of "hyperspaces" and indicate how these spaces interweave the various sciences and practices into a Rainbow Medicine paradigm.

"Inner" and "Outer" Timing

Most people assume that consensus reality—that is, the world of human contacts, linear time, space, and matter—is more significant than dreams and the experience of tendencies. Perhaps you can recall speaking of a dream you've had as though it were imaginary, even though these "imaginary" dreaming spaces and times can be terrifyingly or ecstatically "real." The transition between the various worlds and dimensions is sometimes confusing. For example, someone coming out of a comatose state speaks as if in a dream. Medical helpers are likely to consider ongoing dreamy communication as a pathological event.

The body's subjective experiences, like most internal experiences, have a different timing from the speed of the consensual—the speed at which clocks move. You can feel the difference. When your everyday mind pushes your dreaming body in ways it does not want to go, the body creates a kind of stress reaction, an inner rebellion against everyday time.

If following chronological time brings you too far from body-timing or proprioceptive time, the form of your rebellion may be called a "cold" or "flu." In contrast to an ordinary state of mind, in a Taoist state of mind, the doings of reality and the experiences of the dreaming body come together in a seamless manner. The Tao reminds me of the ancient Greek concept of *kairos*.

In ancient Greece (as well as in other parts of the world), fisherwomen and men gathered each morning on the docks and considered, over coffee, if the *kairos*—that is, the right moment—had come to go fishing. To perceive *kairos* was to perceive the weather and irrational experiences as a source of guidance in determining the presence or absence of propitious circumstances. If the *kairos* was present, fishermen and fisherwomen would go to work. In those days and in that country, *kairos*—in essence, multidimensional perception—was part of consensus reality. Today, consensus reality means following the god of linear time, Kronos: "Make a chronological date, and keep it, whether or not your body agrees!"

These two types of time that we associate with reality and nonconsensus reality, *kronos* and *kairos,* exist side by side. *Kairos* time is like sentient experience or body time. It is neither better nor worse than chronological time; it is simply a "hyperspace," that is, another space beyond the familiar three or four dimensions of everyday life.

What I refer to as Rainbow Medicine lifestyles support awareness of different realities, spaces, and times. Training your awareness to enter dreamlike states, becoming more "lucid," enables you to notice, experience, and follow your subtlest body states while appreciating the everyday world. With training to affirm what you experience, life becomes full of multiple realities. Lucidity and everyday consciousness allow you to understand the consensus reality dimensions of a symptom—the pressure, the change in your body's temperature—while simultaneously experiencing other dimensions—perhaps the dream-state "monsters" and "ghosts" or special powers and subtle feelings. In this way, for example, you may have a pounding headache and simultaneously visualize a dancing drummer creating "pounding," getting you to relax and go into a trance. The trance state is a hyperspace that may resolve the headache. In this way, a symptom may be its own medicine. Said differently, hyperspaces resolve problems in ordinary space and time.

Higher dimensions—hyperspaces—are important for psychology and medicine. We think about and identify ourselves usually as only three-dimensional beings. We do not even have a four-dimensional picture of ourselves, because if we did, we would see ourselves as a moving process, extending throughout time and space. Instead of looking in the mirror to see what we look like, we would say, oh, that mirror is ridiculous. It only gives me a three-dimensional view of myself. I am four-dimensional! I am not the image I see at one time and in one place.

How Hyperspaces Resolve Problems

Today's view of CR is three- or four-dimensional (length, height, width, and time). It's hard to illustrate four dimensions on a two-dimensional surface such as a piece of paper. For a moment, let me simplify the three-dimensional CR into only two dimensions, breadth and length. We are squashing CR a bit for the purpose of explanation. Now CR is like a piece of paper. There is no height in this "Flatland," because CR is now two-dimensional.

Our two-dimensional Flatland reality has no up or down. Imagine that you live in this land and are driving a car (it would have to be very flat car!) from left to right, and meet a barrier, a straight line. If the barrier is not too long, you could drive around it to get to the other side of the barrier.

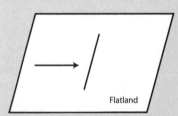

Figure 4-1.

However, if the barrier is very long, then when you got to the barrier, you would not be able to get around it. You would be stuck. In other words, living in Flatland is limiting. When you get stuck, you are simply stuck!

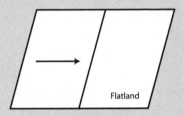

Figure 4-2.

Now imagine good fortune comes your way, and a being from another universe arrives in Flatland and introduces you to a new dimension called height. Adding this new dimension allows new possibilities. Now you can experience going up and down, and soon you discover you can get over the two-dimensional barrier by rising above it. All you needed was an extra dimension to solve the problem.

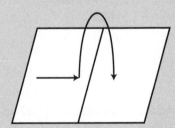

Figure 4-3.

If you lived in Flatland, *height* would be a hyperspace. In the same way, we normally live as if we were Flatlanders. Of course, life on Earth is more than two dimensions; it is three or four dimensions (if you include time). I use Flatland only as an easily imaginable analogy to give you the following idea:

Adding another dimension to your normal world, your everyday space (which is three dimensions) and time (which is the fourth), is to enter a hyperspace. *Hyperspaces solve problems that were impossible in "realities" consisting of fewer spaces*. For example, letting a pounding headache take you into the experience of the pounding beat of a healer's drum is to enter a hyperspace that exceeds four dimensions. The pounding headache is a symptom or event in everyday reality, while the healer's drum is occurring in a hyperspace.

Mathematicians and physicists consider any space beyond three or four dimensions to be a hyperspace. Adding dimensions to CR creates solutions we did not think were possible. Added dimensions help scientists to create a higher-dimensional universe.[2] Likewise, Rainbow Medicine helps to bring in the dreaming dimensions to "real" (CR) symptoms.

If we could find a four-dimensional mirror, we would perhaps see a long, gooey image, including our existence as stardust, previous human lives, our first baby picture, our moment of death, and so forth. In a 2-D mirror, we see instead only a momentary bunch of pimples and wrinkles, and ignore the time and dreamland aspects of ourselves.

A two- or three-dimensional perspective is usually sufficient for most purposes in life, but many problems need more dimensions to get resolved. In a hyperspatial view of yourself, you are not dead or alive, healthy or ill, but an ongoing process moving *between* and *through* all these and other states as well. At any given place, we can be both dead and alive!

Without calling them such, depth psychologists always use hyperspaces. That is why we ask about dreams when clients get blocked. Dreams are a type of hyperspace, which, when added to CR, gives it a new fantasy dimension that offers a way of solving problems that seemed impossible in flat old CR. (Without focusing on CR behavior and cognitive problems, however, even depth psychologists are limited.)

One-color medicine offers Flatland resolutions to multidimensional problems. Have a headache, take an aspirin. If you feel better, think no further about it. However, if the headache returns, it becomes necessary to add dreamland and essence levels.

Jacques Lusseyran and Hyperspaces

One possible reason we ignore hyperspaces is because they may be too small to see. Our eyes do not see little things. For example, at first glance a piece of spaghetti on the floor looks more or less like a straight line to us. However, imagine how a tiny flea might see that same spaghetti. It might feel it was crawling on top of some round world. Likewise, tiny flirts seem small in everyday life only because our normal perception is not trained in picking up the twinklings of nano-level realities. In dreams, however, such flirts can become entire worlds.

In other words, hyperspaces are right here, next to ordinary spaces, or even parallel to them. This idea of the omnipresence of hyperspaces such as dreamland is strongly suggested in the wonderful autobiography of the blind freedom fighter, Jacques Lusseyran. In his book *And There Was Light*, Lusseyran tells how, physically blinded at the age of eight, he developed his awareness of the dreamland universes where images and flirt-like perceptions are possible.[3] After the accident causing his blindness in childhood, he developed a new kind of "seeing": "Now my ears heard the sounds almost before they were there. . . . Often I seemed to hear people speak before they began talking."

He goes on to say that before we touch something, it touches us first. "As your intent to touch arises, you realize that 'it' is actually touching you,"[4] he wrote.

You and the object you relate to are intimate, connected in a nondualistic world. Whereas you might normally think, "I am going to pick up that vase," from the more sentient world of quantum psychology, it is not *you* who does the moving, but rather a coming-together is occurring. Better yet, in a lucid state, you feel that you are both yourself and the object toward which you move.

In Taoism, the "Tao that cannot be said" is said to precede existence, even God. For example, chapter 25 of the *Tao Te Ching* tells us:

> There was something nebulous existing
> Born before Heaven and Earth.
> Silent, empty,
> Standing alone, altering not
> Moving cyclically without becoming exhausted
> Which may be called the mother of all under Heaven.[5]

The realm of the Tao is a hyperspace, the world that can be sensed but not measured or expressed exactly in words.

Exercise: Shape-Shifting

Let's experiment with how engaging your body's hyperspaces can help you resolve any so-called symptoms. In the exercise that follows, I ask that you use your awareness to shape-shift into different forms and other dimensions, as shamans have done in the past. Perhaps children know best about shape-shifting. They don't just play a role; they put on a mask and actually become that role and live in its world for short periods of time.

Sit or lie comfortably. If possible, let your everyday mind relax. Take a few breaths and feel your body.

When you are ready, let your attention gently explore your body. Scan your head, shoulders, chest, midsection, pelvis, legs, feet, and so on.

See, feel, or hear your body. Take note of some subtle sensation that catches your attention which you have not noticed before.

Notice any flickering pressure, heaviness, tremor, pain, burning, and so on. Notice subtle signals, such as slight pressures, sensations, sounds inside your body.

Let your full awareness and attention go to that sensation. Is this sensation possibly connected to a body symptom or one which you fear?

Now, become lucid and catch that sensation. Hold it in your mind's eye, even if it's like a slippery fish that tries to swim away.

Focus on it, or focus on your memory of it. Notice what it looks, feels, or sounds like. Amplify its appearance, feeling, or sound a little bit. Slightly intensify and feel that experience a bit more. Sometimes it helps to use your breath to focus on what you notice, breathing in such a manner that your breath "focuses" on that sensation. Get a good sense of it.

Now use one of your hands to make motions that somehow express what you are experiencing. When you are able to express the inner experiences you are having, ask yourself: "What are my hands expressing?" Here you must trust your inner experience, even it is irrational.

Now, while you are making these hand motions, find out the original impulse behind these motions. To find the "seed" of this experience, it might help you to make the same hand motions again, but while feeling the same intensity, make the motions less and less overt and more and more subtle, until you get a sense of their essence.

Get in touch with the very first tendency behind that hand motion, appearance, feeling, or sound. You may find that it seems to be irrational. Whatever it is, try to believe in it. Focus on that essence, that original tendency, the seed of which gave rise to your body experience. Imagine or experience the basic tendency, intention, motivation, or energy behind the sensation on which you are focusing.

Let your mind express that essence as a sound or as an image. If you get both a sound and an image, try both making the sound and seeing the image at the same time—the sound and the image of the essence of the energy you felt.

In what manner is the world of this sound, this image, this essence, known to you—and yet, at the same time, different from your ordinary world?

What are time and space of the world of this sound/image like? Be a shaman and shape-shift into that image in its world. Take a moment and live in this hyperspace.

If you ignore this world in your everyday life, ask yourself why. Is it too subtle, new, unknown? How could you use this world or incorporate it into the one with which you are more familiar?

Imagine yourself incorporating this new hyperspace. What might you be like?

Make a note of the essence you experienced. Try now to imagine living in this hyperspace. Live in its world, in the time and space of the essence.

Feel how living in this world changes your body experience. If this new hyperspace was originally linked to your experience of body sensations, were those sensations connected to possible symptoms? Living in the essence world, the hyperspace behind those sensations could be very helpful in dealing with those symptoms.

What do you need to feel or do to incorporate this hyperspace into your everyday world?

For example, one woman who had heart problems felt a burning and pulsing sensation in her chest when she first scanned her body. The essence of this burning sensation was a kind of "spark" for her, a tiny and delicate "life impulse." She told me that to live in that space meant for her to "become much more aware of slight sensations" which her "strong and willful nature rarely admitted."

Your Symptom's Spaces

In this exercise, you may have noticed several body dimensions, worlds, or hyperspaces. As the subtle essence experience arises, it flirts with your attention. It appears as a slight sensation, wiggle, thought, or pulse-like form in the essence dimension. You can imagine how, if ignored, this essence experience of the force of silence can become a perception, feeling, or dream image in dreamland. Finally, if this is ignored, it may eventually appear as a visible signal or noticeable symptom.

The body's hyperspaces are where events such as creative urges or symptoms begin. If you are lucid, you won't marginalize subtle experiences and the worlds onto which they open, and symptoms will not have to catch your attention and remind you of what you have ignored. By noticing these spaces, your body symptoms may be relieved, and best of all, your lifestyle can be more creative, even fun.

5 Shamanism and the Essence of Symptoms

I can safely say that nobody understands quantum mechanics. So do not take the lecture too seriously, feeling that you really have to understand in terms of some model . . . but just relax and enjoy it. I am going to tell you what nature behaves like. If you will simply admit that maybe she does behave like this, you will find her a delightful entrancing thing.

—*Richard Feynman[1]*

In this quote, if we replace Feynman's term "quantum mechanics" with the "the force of silence," we move from physics to Rainbow Medicine. Then I can reformulate his words:

We can safely say that nobody understands the force of silence, and you should not feel you have to understand it either. Rather, just relax and enjoy. You will discover for yourself how nature behaves. If you simply admit that She is the way you experience Her, you will find Her a delightful and entrancing hyperspace.

As discussed so far, the earliest stages of awareness—the quantum world's tendencies—are, in essence, a force of silence. At first you only notice a tiny sensation. At this level, there is no difference between fantasies, creativity, matter, psyche, inside, or outside. You just notice the arising of signals and symptoms and the rest of life. Marginalizing this awareness makes you think of yourself in terms of being a body in three dimensions and as having dis-eases or symptoms. When you use your lucid awareness, your life becomes more creative and, to use Feynman's word, an "entrancing" hyperspace.

Training awareness is like training any other capacity: You usually need some instruction and some practice to develop the skill. However, unlike other types of training, you are training yourself to use your awareness in a way that opens you to many worlds at the same time. In my earlier book, *Shaman's Body,* I wrote at length about the particular type of awareness needed for this work. That book is my interpretation of the dazzling shaman, don Juan Matus, the teacher so admirably reported on by the anthropologist Carlos Castaneda.

In the first chapter of *Shaman's Body,* I talked about the courage to facilitate the process of dreaming. In a way, it is a task without end. Only your own body experience and dreams measure your success at this work. Perhaps that is why shamans around the world test their apprentices by exploring their dreams, any illnesses they may undergo, and their ecstatic experiences.[2] These experiences validate the path they are on and tell them what they need to do next.

To me, the existence of symptoms is like a big dream indicating that we are being "called" to undertake a new kind of training. The skills you might need for this training cannot be learned through effort alone, and each situation you meet within yourself seems different or even more impossibly obscure than the last. Perennial philosophies recommend that the best choice for explorers of wisdom at this point is humility. At any degree of accomplishment, you are always a beginner.

Skills can be learned in shamanism and Rainbow Medicine, but they require years of practice to become part of you. During your self-training, you will likely doubt your abilities, perhaps repeatedly. One reason for this recurring disbelief is that fate is always changing what is presented to you. Symptoms remain or change their nature, despite your hard work. The job seems complex and full of inexplicable forces. The idea of controlling our lives with our everyday minds needs to be reframed and infused with the feeling of following nature as a companion. Know that at any point in your work the thing that makes you feel most insecure is insufficient contact with the force of silence.

The shaman understands that what seem to be challenging acts of fate in CR—symptoms, for instance—are not opponents to be overcome but potential allies. Whether the inexplicable forces appear to be monsters or divinities, body problems, world or relationship troubles, they challenge you to expand your identity and learn to move into hyperspaces. One aspect of these powers tempts us to name them, while another aspect of their power avoids everyday descriptions.

Training in Symptom Hyperspaces

Both physics and shamanism helped me understand and approach symptoms in a multidimensional way. Before we begin to work on a symptom in the next pages, let me empathize with the everyday you who suffers from symptoms and perhaps is shy or afraid to work on them. Of course, too much empathy about symptoms can belittle the power in them and invalidate the potential abilities embedded in the trouble.

If you have studied your inner experiences a great deal, meditated, or worked on yourself, you may be reluctant to focus on a symptom, especially if it is chronic, painful, or scary. You may feel you already focus on it too much and are bored or frustrated with it. However, the following innerwork method goes beyond troublesome experiences into possibly unknown hyperspaces. Have the attitude of a shaman's apprentice: Look forward to learning how to use your awareness at different levels of experience, exploring other realms, other worlds. Have courage, but even more importantly, consider the work as an awareness training.

Give yourself time to focus and turn your attention toward your experience. You can do the following exercise either alone or with someone. You will find examples and descriptions of other people's experiences in the parentheses. If these help you to get started, read them; if you prefer a "virgin voyage," just ignore them.

Exercise: Basic Symptom Work

Ask yourself to consider a difficult symptom to focus on. Possibly one you have already thought about, but preferably a symptom you can feel now or one you felt in the past but never understood. By "difficult," I mean choose a symptom that troubles you or makes you afraid. (For example, one of my readers chose to work on a constant sense of bladder pressure.)

With or without the help of a partner, focus on the feeling of that symptom. Put your attention on it and try to feel the sensations of the symptom so exactly that you could recreate it in or on someone else's body, or on a body made of clay, whichever you are more comfortable imagining. Make your description enactment of the symptom so realistic that anyone could experience it. (My reader said that the bladder pressure felt as if something were pushing itself out, against and through the walls of the bladder.)

Do not focus only on the effect the symptom has on you. Focus also on your experience, on your imagination of the energy creating that symptom. This aspect of the exercise might seem very irrational. Nevertheless, use your awareness and catch this dreamlike experience and remember it. (For example: Say you have a headache that is like a sharp pain that makes you feel tired. Do not focus on the tired part that is the effect. Focus instead upon the initial energy or the sharpness of the headache.)

Now unfold the energy behind the symptom by mimicking and expressing its action with one of your hands. This movement may lead you into what I call the "symptom creator," the dreamland predecessor to the physical symptom. Explore shape-shifting into the dreaming realm, and feel and move like that symptom creator until an image emerges of the movement experience. Make a sound that goes with that movement.

Still shape-shifting into that image of the symptom creator, take courage and determine what your sounds and movement are expressing. What is their message? What's in the mind of the symptom creator? Become aware of your experiences.

We are working in a nonconsensual hyperspace, in dreamland. You will have to catch, and believe in, your experiences yourself. There will be no consensus on what you are experiencing. Your own experience is your inner reality.

(My reader with the bladder pressure said: "This pressure feels like a little demon trying to get free. There is a wall, a prison, keeping it in. Some spirit wants to get free.")

Now find the essence of the symptom. To do this, shape-shift into the energy or action of the symptom creator, and begin to move less and still less, all the while feeling the same energy. Then ask yourself to name the essence of the symptom creator. (My reader told me that he moved his hands up against a wall and pressed. But before pressing, before getting so upset, the "demon" was simply a sensitivity to confinement and an urge to be free.)

Once you have found the essence, make an image out of it. This image may be very different from others you have had. This difference should be expected, as we are now moving from dreamland into the essence world. When you can see the essence, move into its world. (My reader said the world was one of delicate flowers.)

What are the time and space of that essence's world like? What does it feel like to be in that world? Live there now. (My reader said the world of flowers had no sense of space, but of freedom, and time was the sense of natural changes from day to night, or season to season.)

Shape-shift and explore the world of the essence. Let your experience express itself in terms of sound, hand movements, perhaps dance-like movements, a quick sketch, or all of these methods. Think of yourself as living art, as a moving sculpture that the force of silence is creating. Keep your focus intense, and let your fantasy unfold until it explains itself to you. (My reader said that this world made him write, that flowers, sun, and a gentle wind caressed his chin. The flowers said, "Slow down, man, you will grow more rapidly."

Someone who suffered from a racing heart and anxiety found that, at first, before the accelerated heart response that was disturbing, there was a sensitivity to a given moment, which appeared as a wisdom teacher who spoke truths.)

Take your time with all this. When you are ready, ask yourself, "How might this experience influence my daily life, my body feelings, my posture, my eating, the way I use my body?" Imagine experiencing the essence of this symptom at home, at work, and in your relationships with others. (For example, the experience might make you more sensitive with your body, more aware and awake to the posture you use when standing and sitting. The way you eat might be changed. If you live in the hyperspace of the symptom, your life at home and work will change, and your relationship problems might become easier to deal with.)

How has this experience already tried to appear in your life? Onto whom or what have you projected the experience? (The reader with the bladder pressure said that he projected the sensitivity onto flowers—he loved to buy flowers—and onto other men who were "like flowers.")

From the world of this experience, feel what is needed to care for your body. What is the essence's "medicine"? The answer to this question is something only you can feel from this space. Focus your attention until you notice the answer from your body wisdom. (My reader was clear: He needed to spend more time in the world of flowers and decided to create a meditation ritual involving his flowers. Also, he was overweight and felt he needed to be lighter and freer.)

Sense how the symptom contains "medicine," not only for itself but also for your life as a whole.

Awareness Practice

When you work on your symptoms, don't just try to heal them. Focus on learning about their unknown inner realms and on awareness practice, experimenting with using your awareness in different ways.

Coming to a particular conclusion or insight is helpful and interesting, but what usually influences symptoms the most is *the awareness practice itself*—your access to your own hyper-spaces, your expanded sense of reality. Developing moment-to-moment awareness leads you toward an increasingly congruent lifestyle. You become more of who you are.

Practice transforms your everyday world into a new kind of space and time. By living closer to the essence of the symptom, you touch its quantum level, its invisible dimensions.

Working with Yourself and Others

In working with yourself or another person using Rainbow Medicine methods, appreciate the CR viewpoint about a given symptom and consider the quantum-physical possibility that you yourself are not located only in your body. Shamans notice that what is happening is not confined to a given locality in time and space. If you work with another person, your feelings and moods are also part of the overall scene. In Rainbow Medicine, there is no well-defined doctor or helper, and no easily identified patient or client. If someone you are helping is blocked, use your own experiences of being blocked. Notice your partner's feedback as she joins you in that experience or in changing it according to her own.

If you are close to the essence level of experience, you may sense what others are going to do before they do anything. The most helpful feeling for working with another person is that you are sharing experiences with him. In fact, it may even sometimes seem as if you know the other person's whole life situation, even if you don't know him well.

A particular shape-shifting event comes to mind. I worked with someone who was suffering from a backache. He described the symptom creator as an "irritant" that made his back muscles cramp. The irritant was so disturbing to my client's conscious mind that he refused to feel any of his back pain. Therefore, instead of asking him to use his awareness to focus on that process, I went into the irritant for him. I became the irritant and made scratching motions in the air. As the irritant, I was so upset I warned my client I could scream.

Suddenly my client admitted to "also" being furious about things. Before my client could say more, I went to the essence of the fury and simply said the word "no" (without knowing quite what I meant). "No," I said, "instead of getting furious, let me say very early on, simply, 'No, I won't, I do not want to'"—still without knowing exactly what I meant. My client burst out laughing, admitting that "no" was a word forbidden for him to say. "No" was often what he felt but never said.

Just talking about the word *no* seemed to relax my client's back muscles. He was very appreciative and liked me so much that he shyly asked if he could spend more private time with me. After a moment of inner turmoil, I managed to say, loudly, "No!"—and we both laughed till tears came to our eyes.

6 What Is Life?

> . . . it has been found that if a vacuum (that is to say, empty space) is compressed, particles appear where there were none before, matter being apparently inherent in some way. These findings would appear to offer an area of convergence between science and the Buddhist "Madhyamika" "theory of Emptiness."
> —His Holiness, the 14th Dalai Lama[1]

Life seems to pop up from nothing; events arise out of the blue. Quantum physics and spiritual traditions almost agree on this. Shamans tap into the life force of silence, finding Rainbow Medicine from nano-level body sensations and hyperspaces. In this chapter, I explore ideas about life as described in biology and biophysics. In the next chapter I combine ideas from spiritual traditions, shamanism, and quantum physics with those from biology. A new picture of human beings emerges with this synthesis.

In physics and medicine, our CR definition of ourselves is based upon marginalization of dreamland and essence worlds. In the new paradigm, there is a shift in the "assemblage point," as the shaman don Juan says. Your "assemblage point" is the way in which you "assemble" or identify yourself. If you consider yourself a real point, your assemblage point will be in consensus reality. If you identify yourself as an awareness focuser, your assemblage point will span the various levels of dreaming and reality. In terms of the present work, this means that our identity is no longer identical with consensus reality but includes the experience of the force of silence that gives rise to all the other worlds.

In the Rainbow Medicine paradigm, the human being is both real (a physical body) and a quantum wave (a tendency or intentional wave experience). First we are an essence, an intent, unfolding into the forms of dreamland, which then informs us of probable identities in CR. We choose one of these and call it our human form. In the new paradigm, all events are multidimensional. Everything viewed in CR as unintentional, e.g., as a problem or a disease becomes a sign of wholeness in Rainbow Medicine.

In the new paradigm dis-ease is a sign of the mystery of life, the means by which new and unidentified forms of life can emerge. If you shift your assemblage point and experience the hyperspace of the tendencies, you become aware of your nonlocal form, an intent that manifests in many ways including your bodily form in CR.

Theoretical Viewpoints on the Origins of Life

Every physical object in our universe is multidimensional, "entangled" with everything around it. Today's biology, however, often speaks about life only in terms of CR dimensions. Without hyperspatial thinking that includes the world of nonlocal quantum mechanics, a clear, local, body-oriented definition of life is difficult to create.

Astronomers and biologists believe life began on Earth about three billion years ago. According to some scientific theories and evidence, the origins of the universe occurred with a Big Bang, 18 billion years ago. If cosmologists are right, our Earth and solar system were formed roughly five billion years ago. Research shows that consensual forms of life first appeared on Earth around three billion years ago. No one knows for sure how the complexity called "life" arose. What makes a group of chemicals suddenly combine in such a manner to form a living being?

Quantum mechanics does not have a firm answer, though we know that according to quantum theory, material particles "pop up" out of nothing, that is, out of a vacuum, out of so-called zero-point energy states. Buddhism thinks similarly, but calls the state "emptiness." In the quote from the Dalai Lama at the beginning of the chapter, he states that matter and perhaps life itself are "inherent" in the nondualistic, nonlocal world of the essence.

To use the "powers" of the shaman in order to "merge with the night" and move through the darkness, don Juan tells his apprentices to feel the environment. This feeling is similar to the nonlocal interconnectedness or life experience connecting observer and observed that Jacques Lusseyran describes after being blinded at the age of eight. Describing how he sensed a tabletop, he says:

> To find out, my fingers had to bear down, and the amazing thing is that the pressure was answered by the table at once. Being blind I thought I should have to go out to meet things, but I found that they came to me instead. . . . I didn't know if I was touching [an apple] or it was touching me. As I became part of the apple, the apple became part of me . . . everything was an exchange of pressures. . . . I spent hours leaning against objects and letting them lean against me.[2]

Without our normal ability to see, we must use "hypersenses" to detect the hyperspaces we typically marginalize in daily life. When "seeing" instead of "looking," we feel life to be entangled with everything around us. As Lusseyran said, "I didn't know if I was touching [an apple] or if it was touching me."[3] This reminds me of John Cramer's description of the quantum world characterized by "reflected waves" or what I call co-reflective impulses.[4] At the deepest level, we can't tell if we are senders or receivers of signals and experiences.

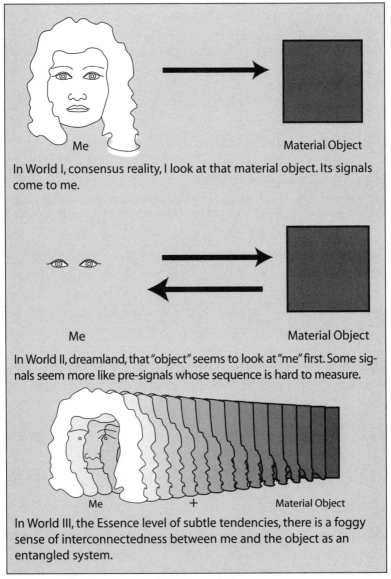

In World I, consensus reality, I look at that material object. Its signals come to me.

In World II, dreamland, that "object" seems to look at "me" first. Some signals seem more like pre-signals whose sequence is hard to measure.

In World III, the Essence level of subtle tendencies, there is a foggy sense of interconnectedness between me and the object as an entangled system.

Figure 6-1. Multidimensional Experiences of Matter

Physicists on Mind and Matter

In the diagram, World III, the Essence Level world—what the Dalai Lama refers to as "emptiness"—seems to me to refer to what some physicists and Jack Sarfatti and David Bohm refer to as the quantum wave function. World III experiences seem as if they have foggy undifferentiated content. Sarfatti quotes David Bohm as speaking about quantum waves as "thought-like" experiences. Physicists Fritjof Capra[6] and Fred Alan Wolf[7] also refer to the mind's quantum-realm features and connect physics to Buddhist and other spiritual teachings.

Perception and awareness may not be located only inside of us.[5] I suggest that the source of life itself does not reside within any particular body, but is a shared, entangled experience involving all of us, the environment, and anything and everything in the universe.

In consensus reality, you may be concerned with "your" life. However, with expanded awareness, life turns out to be a shared process, continuously unfolding flirts from multiple locations.

From experiential and theoretical viewpoints, from Buddhism and physics, life may be considered a CR fact *and* an immeasurable dreamland experience. Judging from the original meaning of the word *life,* our ancestors apparently knew that life and "tendencies" are connected. In Merriam-Webster's dictionary, life is connected with "energy," "vivacity," "spark," and *"the tendency to react."*

Life in Biology

Biology focuses mainly on the parameters of consensus reality in defining life. In the *Encyclopedia Britannica (2002)* under "Definitions of Life," we find various examples. One is: "Living systems [demonstrate] the ability to take in food, adapt to the environment, grow, and reproduce offspring." The biological definition of life found in physiological systems theory is: "A system is alive if it metabolizes." The metabolic definition of life

Evolution and Genetics

In his famous book, *Origin of the Species* (1859), Darwin spoke of the great battle he called "survival of the fittest." This phrase means if we adapt to our environment better than our peers, we are more likely to live than they. According to the basic genetic theory of evolution, we reproduce because our genes, which are encoded within our DNA, split and form new cells. If you mate with someone of the opposite sex, your genes mix together, creating a new person. If the new person mates with someone, again the genes mix. Sometimes mutations occur, and a gene gets "broken" or otherwise changed.

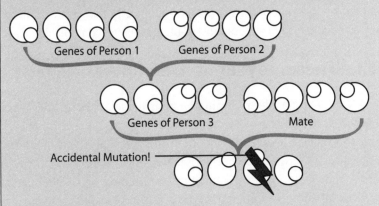

In this diagram the genes of Persons 1 and 2 come together and produce a new person. The new person meets someone else and they reproduce, but at the bottom of the picture we see that one of the genes changes unpredictably because of some mutation.

According to Darwin's theory, if the mutated person is "fit" she survives; otherwise, she dies. It turns out that most mutations are losers in this fateful game and produce "unfit" life forms.

Figure 6-2. Mutation

includes identity. A system is alive if it has "a definite boundary and exchanges material with the outside but remains itself over time."

These CR definitions are problematic. A car has a boundary, and it might be thought of as "metabolizing" gas-food, yet most would deny that it is "alive." In biochemistry, a system is alive if it "reproduces, carries hereditary information encoded in nucleic acid molecules, and metabolizes using enzymes."[8]

Medical or biological theories based upon evolutionary theories mirror our CR psychology that discards experiences deemed unfit or inappropriate.[9] This kind of thinking leads to cultural unconsciousness and xenophobia. Marginalizing parts of ourselves leads to diversity problems, wherein we belittle histories if they don't "fit" in with the "norm." Unbeknownst to us, the more we marginalize others, the more terrified of ourselves we become. Anxieties of all kinds are linked to having ignored part of ourselves, or ignoring outer worlds as well. In other words, evolutionary theory merely reflects our problematic everyday psychology.

The Thermodynamic Definition of Life

Now let's consider thermodynamical ideas about life. Local biological definitions of life are extended by the physics of energy transfer, which describes life in terms of shared cosmological energies. According to thermodynamics, our lives are a form of order that depends on the life and eventual death of the sun, as well as all the other energy sources around us. Life comes from the neg-entropy of energy sources such as the sun. In a way, stars die so that we can live. As we live, eventually our bodies' order becomes disorderly and, with "death," turns to dust—which, in turn, nourishes other life forms. Using concepts of entropy and energy supports the idea of life as interdependent phenomena. All life on Earth is linked cosmologically with the energy of stars.

The Rainbow View of Life

In the Rainbow Medicine view of life, everything in the universe is "alive" in dreamland and part of the life process. Your experience of interdependent flickers and flirts indicates that life is properly shared with the whole universe. In dreamland and hyperspaces, objects and people are all vivacious, whether they live or appear "dead" in consensus reality.[10]

Thermodynamics

Thermodynamics, the theory of the transfer of energy and matter, determines the processes in the macroscopic world.

All usable energy, such as that comprising CR notions of life, is a form of what physicists call "neg-entropy." Entropy is a form of disorder. Life, simply stated, is a form of order or neg-entropy. When systems lose their order or neg-entropy, they dissolve or die. On Earth, our main source of neg-entropy is the sun. Thus the origins of life on Earth are tied up with sources of neg-entropy and usable energy from the sun. In the diagram, the sun feeds our Earth. Our bodies on Earth gain life, in part, from the sun.

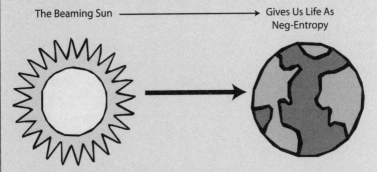

The Beaming Sun ⟶ Gives Us Life As Neg-Entropy

The sun beams neg-entropy to us. However, in the overall balance of things, every sunbeam we get from the sun costs the sun some energy and "life."

Figure 6-3. The Beaming Sun Gives Us Life As Neg-Entropy

The phenomenon of *life* is a multidimensional reality requiring both consensual and hyperspatial considerations. Life and wellness depend upon CR facts and energy, our genes and sunshine, food and water, as well as quantum-realm experiences. Our sense of life is strongly connected with hyperspaces. If you are lucid about your contact with the force of silence, you feel alive and well. If you are not, you may feel chronically and mildly depressed and uncreative. Then instead of new flirts and sparkles popping up, your attention is drawn toward symptoms and ascertaining your degree of bodily health or illness.

It sometimes seems to me as if life were a kind of fairy-tale figure who transforms from a good fairy into a jealous monster, saying, "Don't ignore me! Give me every creative moment, notice the little flickers, or I will create something that forces you to admit to my (and your) creativity!"

If one-color medicine's job is to preserve life, then Rainbow Medicine's job is to arouse awareness to cull the intention of symptoms and everything that catches our attention. Life is the creativity of the moment. Like one-color medicine, Rainbow Medicine aims at curing symptoms. But unlike one-color medicine, the new paradigm also welcomes dis-ease and deals with illness at many levels, seeing disease and aging as new forms of creativity.

7 The Ghost of Atoms

Aborigine creation myths tell of legendary
totemic beings who had wandered over every
continent in the Dreamtime, singing out the
name of everything that crossed their path—
birds, animals, plants, rocks, waterholes—and so
singing, the world came into existence.
—*Bruce Chatwin,*[1] The Songlines

In his 1987 book *The Songlines,* Bruce Chatwin tells how the
Aboriginal person must know the sacred song of an area to travel
through life. People have always believed that singing songs in
altered states of consciousness changes the world. According to
our Aboriginal ancestors, what I am calling the force of silence
they might call the Great Spirit that forms the Earth, transforming
geology into sacred territory.

Songs, the feeling of music, and waves guide life into being. If
we are to judge by the work of some of the most renowned and
controversial scientists, such as David Bohm, physics may be trying to catch up to these ancient ideas. In chapter 2, I discussed

Bohm's idea that quantum waves contain/are nonconsensual information—in his words, "pilot waves" leading objects about as if they (the waves) had some sort of inner wisdom. Aboriginal dreaming and Bohm's "pilot waves" are what we might call "the ghosts of the atoms" that move our bodies.

Entelechy—Ideas of a Guiding Force

The idea that a guiding force appears in both living and so-called inanimate matter has been proposed by many. The Greek philosopher Aristotle thought life was a force that gives organisms their properties.[2] Moreover, he saw the whole cosmos as an organism that could not be divided up into parts. The modern theoretical physicist Paul Davies points out in his book *The Fifth Miracle* that science has largely discredited older notions of life as a guiding vitalist force.[3] This is an elusive, immeasurable factor in matter that is supposed to have created life and which moves along with material bodies informing them about their path.

Yet this idea of a mystical force could never be repressed. In the nineteenth century, for example, after electricity was discovered, Mary Shelley created her fantastic figure of Frankenstein, showing that vitalism, as a philosophy, was still alive. In her tale, the imaginary figure called Frankenstein brought his "monster" to life by a vitalistic bolt of lightning from a thunderstorm.

The idea of a guiding force has always been part of humankind's thinking. Gottfried Wilhelm Leibniz, the seventeenth-century German philosopher, mathematician, and physicist who discovered calculus (concurrently with Newton), called the ultimate reality of material things "monads" or "entelechies"—that is, informing spirits. According to him, all objects possess inner, self-determined life forces. The twentieth-century German biologist Hans Driesch used the concept of entelechy to denote an internal perfecting principle which he proposed existed in all living organisms. This biologist apparently followed in the footsteps of Aristotle and Leibniz, considering entelechy a life-giving force. For him, entelechy was a kind of soul that was responsible for the development of all living things.

Today, the idea of a guiding soul or wave is replaced, by and large, by science's proclamation that the origins of life can be found in a freak accident of chemistry, unique to Earth. Most scientists believe that some special set of chemical, thermodynamic, and electrical circumstances produced the first signs of life in accordance with chance, which rules subsequent evolution. However, in August 1996, some scientists began to reconsider this belief in the uniqueness of life on Earth.

After researching the ancient meteorite that struck our Earth from Mars, evidence was found for life on Mars. Some scientists now believe that life is part of the natural order of the universe and that life came from Mars (while others hypothesize that basic elements of life, such as amino acids, were formed in interstellar space and came to Earth via meteorites).

Similar to Aristotle, Leibniz, and Driesch, physicist Paul Davies believes that the secret of life comes from the invisible, informational properties of matter. As he discusses in *The Fifth Miracle,* he feels these informational properties are located in the wave function. According to Davies, life—that is, the growth and development of organisms with attributes of autonomy, complexity, and reproductive, metabolic, and nutritional capacities— comes from the informational content of a nonlocal global wave function. In other words, the serpentine wave function is another kind of modern "guiding force."

Wave Functions and Kundalini

Focusing on a proposed connection between consciousness and gravity, Oxford cosmologist Roger Penrose, in his book *The Emperor's New Mind,* suggests that gravity affects bio-molecules through quantum processes. In his view, the origin of life is linked with gravity, the curved nature of space, and the origins of the universe.

Many of these new ideas in physics about consciousness and life seem to have roots in the mid-twentieth-century work of David Bohm described in his book *The Undivided*

Universe: An Ontological Interpretation of Quantum Theory. There he explored the roots of physics to explain the unity and nonlocality of the universe that became evident in the first nonlocality experiments.[4] For Bohm, the quantum wave function is an information carrier, continuously interacting with everything around it.

When *any* event occurs, *everything* participates. All the various aspects of the event are interconnected. For example, your wave function describes your relationships with other people, your chair, your cup, and all the things around you as co-creating participants.

David Bohm used the term "pilot wave" to describe the "active" information in the wave function. He imagined the pilot wave as following and guiding particles as they move about. The wave traveled with its objects, leading them about, not totally unlike Aristotle's, Leibniz's, and Driesch's notions of entelechy.

Quantum Waves in Flight

Let us think about what happens to an electron when it is emitted from an electron gun in order to understand the potential meaning of physicists' ideas about quantum waves.

In the diagram "Flight of an Electron," notice three areas: I, II, and III. In area I, the electron (the dark spot) is in a gun just before it is shot through the slit. In area II, though the electron's exact flight path or trajectory cannot be tracked (measured physically) because any measurement would collapse the wave function, we still know that the electron can be represented by a wave (from the quantum wave equation) until it lands at point B in area III—where the electron detector beeps, indicating an electron has arrived.

In this view, the electron is imagined to be a particle in area I, before emission (though its exact nature cannot be seen). In phase II, quantum physics describes the particle as a virtual wave; the mathematical formulation is exact but immeasurable in CR reality.

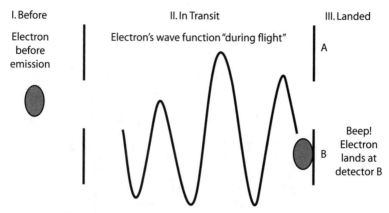

I. Before

Electron before emission

II. In Transit

Electron's wave function "during flight"

III. Landed

A

B

Beep! Electron lands at detector B

Figure 7-1. Flight of an Electron

The concept of the quantum-level wave is an imaginary complex number; it is a dreamland, pulse-like idea, something perhaps thought or felt but not seen or measured. The imaginary characteristics of the wave function gave rise to many analogies in consensus reality. That is why, since the 1920s when quantum physics started to evolve, the discoverer of quantum waves, Erwin Schrödinger, believed they were real "matter waves," as he called them. However, such waves have never been observed in CR experiments.

Apparently Bohm picked up on this early idea about the vibratory quality of the wave function, which had already been proposed, in part, by an earlier quantum physicist, Louis DeBroglie. It was DeBroglie who, in 1923 (as a Sorbonne graduate student), discovered that particles exhibit wavelike properties that describe "certain internal cyclic processes" of the particles. Though future developments in physics showed that "matter waves" were not measurable, some physicists today still refer to Bohm's idea of the "pilot wave."[5]

Bohm argued in *The Undivided Universe* that the wave description of (area II) is as accurate as the mathematics itself: "The imaginative qualitative concept is therefore, in the long run, just as key a feature of this overall appearance [of quantum theory] as is the precise and abstract mathematical concept. The two

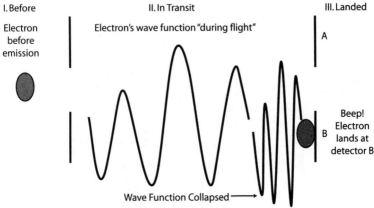

I. Before   II. In Transit   III. Landed

Electron before emission

Electron's wave function "during flight"

A

Beep! Electron lands at detector B

B

Wave Function Collapsed ⟶

Figure 7-2. Nonlocality in Phase II

together not only present a more comprehensive appearance than either one alone could do, but also each can serve as a clue for further development in the other."

Nonlocality

The wave equation represents a nonlocal phenomenon in quantum theory. That is, in its unmeasured states, in area II, the wave representing the particle can be any place at any time in the universe. Only when the "particle" is observed does it "collapse" from its wavelike nature into being particle-like, located in a spot, such as B. See figure 7-2. There is no one accepted scientific explanation for how this occurs; it remains one of quantum mechanics' mysteries (which I have interpreted as being due to marginalization of the subtle background behind everyday events).

In area II, the wave function or pilot wave is nonlocal until "collapsed" by measurement. In its "larger" nonlocal state as the guiding wave, it is anywhere in the universe, and it is connected to everything.

Bohm put the idea of the particle and wave together by imagining the graphic analogy of a ship and a radar wave guiding it. Though in measurable (CR) reality there is no wave or particle

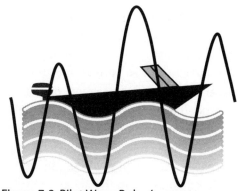

Figure 7-3. Pilot Wave. Bohm's quantum wave pictured as an informational flow guiding a ship at sea.

which can be singularly measured, Bohm used his imagination to explain how a quantum wave could be visualized as guiding the particle with which it is associated. Using the analogy of a ship at sea, he said the particle was like a ship, and the wave function was a radar wave that pilots the ship through the sea. See my picture of his imagination.

In this pictorial analogy, the ship "senses" the waves and guides itself accordingly. Everything that happens on this ship—the thoughts of the captain, the behavior of the crew, the engine's functioning—is interconnected with this pilot wave "intelligence." Such a picture is a combination of consensus reality and dreamland versions of the same thing. The CR version of a particle or object, here symbolized by the ship, is extended by the dreamland imagination of a virtual or mathematical description.

Pilot or Quantum Waves in Rainbow Medicine

In a kind of psychological slang, we might say that every particle and person has a kind of "buzz" or life force. We have well known measurable electromagnetic fields around us, and also immeasurable fields. I would have ignored Bohm's idea of pilot waves as wishful thinking if I had not already experienced something like a pilot wave guiding my own life, as well as the lives of individuals, couples, and groups. After thinking about the many thousands of people I have worked with in my practice and in seminars around the world, and the way my life has unfolded, there is little doubt in my mind that there is a sort of informational wave pattern—a personal myth, relationship myth, or group vision—which moves and guides us through life. If C. G. Jung, the Swiss psychiatrist and founder of the school of analytical psychology that I first attended, were alive today, I am sure he would say, "Of course, the pilot wave is what I called the individual's personal myth!"

I need only think of my early interest in physics, the apparently improbable accidents that landed me in the applied physics area of M.I.T., how my fascination with Einstein drew me to study in Zurich where I landed one week after Jung died in 1961. My first dream of analysis was about Jung telling me to pull together psychology and physics. Finally, after relationship changes, I married Amy, born on the day Jung's main collaborate in physics, the Nobel Prize winner Wolfgang Pauli, had died. Are all these things accidents? I arrived the week Jung died, and Amy "arrived" the day Pauli died.

Even if you never knew what to call it, you too have probably felt, at one time or another, that some sort of repetitive pattern characterizes your life. In terms of our bodies, the "captain" is that part of us who thinks she is steering "her" ship. Many of our problems come from the fact that she, the captain, does not realize that all the things she calls "her" thoughts are coming to her from the much wider expanse of her dreaming. Yet we all know that our lives are not directed entirely by us, but by something that looks like a bunch of accidents and incidental events.

Our pilot waves can be seen in our first memories and childhood dreams, which have piloted us about, more or less predicting what our psychological experience will be. In fact, with expanded awareness, we can become aware, at every moment of the day, that while we inhabit physical bodies, at the same time, there is a kind of intentional field, a buzz around us, that gently moves us in subtle ways but which we usually marginalize. As I have shown before, this marginalization apparently increases its intensity, until it feels like a direct push or pull in reality, and appears in what everyone calls *symptoms*. The threat and power of symptoms might appear in dreams to be a dragon or serpent.

Back Action

Bohm did not believe that the pilot wave entirely determined the particle's/ship's path, but that the behavior of the particle/ship reciprocally influenced the pilot wave. He called this influence "back action." Back action is a kind of feedback between body and mind. To be more exact, it is a non-consensual feedback between the body and awareness and the force of silence.

A psychological analogy of back action is the experience of how changes in your everyday attitude influence the course of your dreams. Back action is crucial to our sense of emotional and psychological balance.

To the everyday mind that is very much out of touch with quantum wave experiences or the force of silence, this energy appears awesome. I think of the kundalini, the creative force, or the Taoist dragon, a yang force.

Once the everyday mind is more in tune with this energy, the fierce dragon transforms, and now looks happier, in the form of the Immortal Taoist who is one with the waves. (See figure 7-4.)

The Immortal Taoist is a picture of what we may look like when we are one with the wave patterns. We mirror the fish in the sea as well as the clouds in the air. After we have "shifted our assemblage point" from the everyday world to the hyperspace of tendencies, the division between the pilot wave and ourselves diminishes until there is no sense of division. In that moment, you don't *do* something; rather you experience it as *getting done*.

Some of us relate better to the mathematics of physics, others to Taoist analogies or Buddhist teachings about *Mu-shin*, which means both "emptiness" and "creative mind." For me, the piloting power of intentional waves is the basis of Rainbow Medicine; it is the force of silence mirrored in the vitalist philosophy still present in physics and projected into the quantum wave concept.

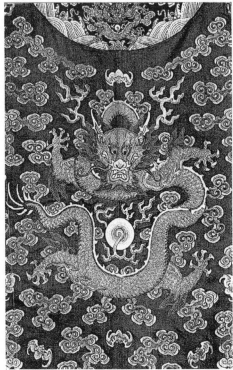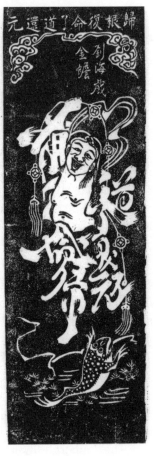

Figure 7-4. Taoist Dragon[6] and Immortal
Taoist[7]. Transformation of pilot wave experience from original form as a dragon to
dancing with waves.

Photo Jeff Teasdale. From *Tao: The Chinese Philosophy
of Time and Change* by Philip Rawson and Laszlo
Legeza, published by Thames & Hudson Inc., New York.

Speculations about this nonconsensual force have located it as

- the origin of life
- *chi* body energy
- the accidental chemistry at the beginning of our world or universe
- the spirit of reproduction, identity, and evolution
- what is present in meteorites from outer space that affects bio-
molecules.

Perhaps it is that part of us that is everywhere and immortal. We are our community, our world, as well. This reminds me of an African proverb, told to me by Dr. John L. Johnson, "I am because you are. And you are because I am." Life does not belong to you or me alone; we live only because of everything else.

The ghost of what we today call atoms was felt and expressed by Aboriginal people through sacred songs, guiding them through unknown territories. In European science, Leibniz suspected such informing spirits existed in all living and so-called inanimate matter. He called them "monads" or "entelechies." In contemporary science, David Bohm and, more recently, Paul Davies and others believe this force can be found in the invisible, informational properties of the wave function.

For me, the piloting power of intentional waves is the quantum source of information and healing. Our lucid awareness of this in-formation gives us subtle, yet direct body experience of the silent force mirrored in vitalist philosophy and present day physics.

8 Parallel Song Worlds

> If we take [Stephen] Hawking seriously, it means
> that we must begin our analysis with an infinite
> number of all possible universes, coexisting with
> one another. To put it bluntly, the definition of the
> word universe is no longer "all that exists." It now
> means "all that can exist."
>
> —*Michio Kaku*[1]

In this chapter I will show how wave theory, Aboriginal songlines, and physics help us understand dreams and body symptoms.

In the preceding chapters, I have suggested that life is a multileveled awareness experience mirrored in the mathematics of
the quantum waves "behind" or "beneath" what we experience as
reality. I suggested that our deepest sense of life is a movement
tendency that can be felt when the ordinary mind is relaxed.
Dreams arise out of those micromovements, or out of the force of
silence, which is symbolized in quantum physics as an object's
wave function. We experience this wave function or intentional

wave directly only as a subtle sense of guidance, as the sense of a personal myth. Since we feel best when we are connected with these tendencies, I refer to the intentional wave as the "path with heart," composed of multiple states and experiences or parallel worlds.

The Pilot Wave's Many Worlds

What I call "the force of silence" is described differently, depending on the awareness level of the person doing the describing.

Consensus Reality: In CR, experimental physics can only measure the most probable aspects of the essence world, the force of silence. As I have said previously, the standard idea of observation marginalizes all the virtual aspects needed to create the CR version of reality, just as looking at a tree can marginalize the importance of its roots. Seen and experienced from the viewpoint of consensus reality, the force of silence appears to be unintentional, accidental—a dreamland image, something that is easily ignored.

Dreamland: In theoretical physics, the force of silence appears as a wave in an imaginary space. (That is, the math of the wave function describes it in a mathematical space of complex numbers.) In dreamland experiences, the force of silence appears as dreams and images in the body, which, averaged over long periods of time, amount to our personal myth.

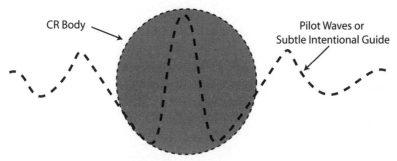

Figure 8-1. The CR You with Your Guiding Pilot Wave

Essence: Though words don't fit this realm, the concepts of the essence and sense of guiding intention point to nondualistic experiences of the force of silence, such as tendencies and flirts. As discussed earlier, Bohm imagined this realm in terms of the pilot wave. The essence lies behind psychology (personal myth), physics (the wave function), and therefore all objects in CR. Putting these various concepts and images together, we come up with the picture in figure 8-1.

Water, Quantum, and Dream Waves

To understand how the pilot wave, or any wave, is composed of many other waves (and many worlds), remember being in a lake or by the seashore. Recall how passing boats disturb existing waves on the water's surface. At any one moment, a boat's wave adds to the existing water waves, making a new wave, which is the sum of the first two (see figure 8-2).

Waves are wonderful![2] The resulting new wave (merely a sketch in the illustration, not mathematically precise) is the sum of the waves the boat makes plus the preexisting wave, which was there before the boat passed. Even more amazing to those of us fascinated by waves is that after the boat is gone and its wave has passed along, the water goes back to its preexisting pattern,

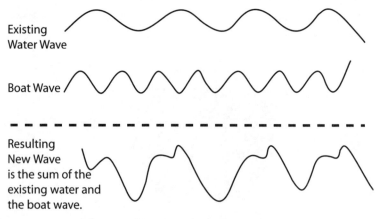

Existing Water Wave

Boat Wave

Resulting New Wave is the sum of the existing water and the boat wave.

Figure 8-2. How Waves Add to One Another

unchanged. In other words, water waves (and waves in general) are more or less independent of one another, especially in a very large body of water like the ocean. They merge with each other, then go their separate ways after the "merger." Each wave is a world unto itself.

We can use these characteristics of waves to connect psychology and physics. We have already considered that particles and material objects such as atoms have pilot or quantum waves and that people have quantum waves or personal myths. The pilot or quantum wave of an atom can be broken down into sub-waves that do not interfere with one another.[3] Each sub-wave represents the manner in which the atom can "vibrate."

Likewise, our basic patterns or personal myths are composed of sub-personalities, which, like waves, usually exist without interfering with one another. Each sub-personality is a pattern of how we can behave; at night, we may dream about various sub-patterns or fragment of dreams. The various sub-personalities or fragments of any one night's dreaming barely seem to interact with one another. We can be a wise woman in one state, and an angry child in another, and the two states barely interact with each other. (That's why we need therapists to help.)

Just as the overall wave of an atom is the sum of its various sub-specific atomic states, so we are a wave resulting from many "boats" at sea. Thus you might consider your various friends and enemies as sub-waves, each in a different world.

Exercise: Sub-Personalities and Music

To understand how you may be the sum of other waves and to understand wave theory better, try the following experiment with yourself.

Choose either a recent dream or a dream from long ago. Remember just one dream with a couple of images in it.
Think of one of the dream figures, "Figure A" in your dream, and try to express that image as a simple sound and rhythm. Don't take long

at this; just think of the figure and make a sound and any rhythm that goes with it, to express that figure. (You may notice that this sound and rhythm give you a hint about the possible meaning of that figure.)

Now do the same with Figure B from that dream. Express the image with another simple sound and rhythm. (You may notice that this sound and rhythm give you a hint about the possible meaning of that figure.)

Finally, experiment with your creativity and put these two sounds/rhythms together. Can you do that? The resulting sound and rhythm—let's call that "sound" Figure C—represent more of the whole of you than either A or B.

The music of Figures A and B are "sub-states" or sub-personalities of the sound C. The final sound C may give you a sense of your overall pattern or momentary "pilot wave."[4]

The sum of all your dream figures across your lifetime is, in a way, your life's pilot wave. The sum of your sub-states more closely represents your overall nature. Musical waves are the same (mathematically) as water and quantum waves. Perhaps this is why physicists such as Einstein, Pauli, and Feynman have been fascinated by music—its sounds, tones, and overtones.

Any wave or any sound (or any experience) contains other waves and sub-waves, other tones and sub-tones (or overtones). Focusing, as we normally do, on only the most obvious tones or parts of our nature marginalizes the sub-tones. If you focus on only one body state—for example, pushing to do something—you will automatically marginalize the deeper states of consciousness that are needed in creating the large "you" and your overall pattern. Choosing to identify only with one part of your overall pilot wave such as "being good" marginalizes the rest of your nature and its "sub-tones."

Musical Tones, Overtones, and Waves

I agree with Richard Feynman that the idea that any wave can be understood as the sum of sub-waves[5] is one of the most amazing theories in all of science. Musicians feel or know about sub-waves or tones. For example, when a single note is played on a piano, we actually hear several tones at once, called *overtones*. Each piano (or guitar, cello, etc.) note is really a rich combination of many pitches. Overtones are often too faint to hear, unless you have trained your musical ear. The overtone is a faint tone that sounds higher (or lower) than the fundamental tone when a string or air column vibrates as a whole.

If you can, pluck the lowest string, the E string, on a guitar. When you pluck that string, you hear the fundamental tone of E. However, if you put your finger gently on the middle of a string, you will notice that the string no longer vibrates as a whole but instead vibrates on both sides of your finger—and the tone is an octave higher. Pluck E and then put your finger in the middle of the string, and you will hear E one octave higher!

Even more exciting is the following discovery (made by the Greeks centuries ago). When you play the fundamental tone again, you can also hear the higher-octave tone as a subtle part of the basic tone. The higher tone is an "overtone" of the base tone. You have discovered that the *string can vibrate in several different ways at the same time.* Like all strings and waves, the

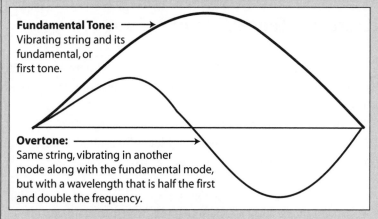

Fundamental Tone: ⟶
Vibrating string and its fundamental, or first tone.

Overtone: ⟶
Same string, vibrating in another mode along with the fundamental mode, but with a wavelength that is half the first and double the frequency.

Figure 8-3. Vibrating String and Its Overtone

tones we hear are a combination of other tones—waves or overtones superimposing upon one another, just as water waves add up, one upon the other.

Overtones are always there; you just need training to hear them. Like the average listener, I normally hear the fundamental pitch clearly, and only with concentration can I hear the faint overtones.

In the diagram, I have drawn the fundamental tone and the first overtone. There are other overtones with more wavelengths, but for simplicity, let's think only about a basic sound containing a basic tone, like the guitar's E, which contains both that E and its overtone. The instrument playing any given E, such as a guitar or piano, has more or less of given overtones.

Without realizing it, we determine whether a guitar or piano is playing that E by unconsciously noticing the particular overtones the instrument produces.

Although the volume of the tone may be the same in each instrument, each overtone has a different strength in each instrument. The different strengths of the mixture tell us we are hearing a trumpet instead of a piano or a voice. Still, because of the strength of the main tone, we can tell that all the notes of the different instruments are playing the same note.

Physicists and mathematicians (and now healers of all sorts as well) know that the overall resulting sounds of things and people are combinations of basic tones and overtones.

Exercise: Tones Express Body

Neglecting one of your sub-states or tones makes you feel incomplete or unwell. To increase your awareness of your everyday self and the hyperspaces you live in at any given moment, ask yourself: What is the fundamental tone I feel? What are its overtones?

Try the following exercise in which I invite you to represent body feelings by sounds and tones.

When you are ready, sense the atmosphere inside and around your body. What tone most clearly represents the body state you are in this moment? Is it sharp, undulating, deep, soft, hard? Make a sound that represents this inner state. Even if you are shy about sounds, make this tone now. Hold it long enough to hear a simple, clear tone.

Next, listen to your particular sound and let yourself fantasize about that sound. Go into its world. Imagine a story line that goes with that sound. This need not be a big story, just a little story. Whatever it is, tell the story. What is the world like in this story of the sound? For example, one reader heard a train and saw himself chugging along, hearing the choo-choo sounds of the locomotive. He fantasized the train was going east, crossing from Russia to China.

When you are ready, raise the tone of that first sound by one octave (or what you think might be an octave higher). This will be the first overtone. Make the overtone sound to yourself so you can hear it. (If it is uncomfortable to sing the higher octave, try one octave below your fundamental sound.)

Hear and feel and sense the overtone's world. What images or story unfolds in the presence of this overtone? Wait for quick, flickering ideas, catch them, and tell a story or fantasy connected to this overtone.

Move and shape-shift. That is, *feel* yourself *into* the world of the overtone, and try living there in your fantasy. Feel it. Sing its sound and tell its story at the same time. Make a note about your experiences of this world. How is it the same or different from the first world?

While you are living in this parallel world, ask yourself: What is its message? How does this message make sense in my ordinary, everyday life? How might this message help with the situations I have been working on? For example, the octave above the choo-choo train sounded to my reader like a high-pitched rocket motor going into outer space. This felt irrational to him, and he had to train himself to accept rather than marginalize that experience. Then he imagined living in that world, in outer space, and it was very different from the state of the first chugging train-like sound. My reader said the message for him was to let himself "float" more instead of moving ahead in an effortful, chugging fashion in life.

Finally, ask yourself: How were the sound and message of the overtone already present within the first tone, but in a way which I did not pay attention to before? My reader associated China, the place his train was heading, as old China, "another world," where, he imagined, Taoists lived who "floated" with life.

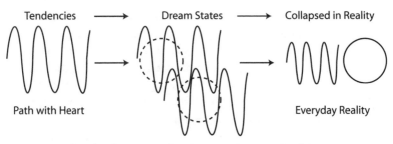

Figure 8-4. Sketch of How Tendencies May Become Realities

Overtones usually seem like "far out" altered states of consciousness. Normally, we live in only one of our many dimensions by focusing only on the first tone, which is best known. This is the one with which we identify most closely. But this world is a one-sided Flatland compared to the hyperspaces of our overtones. In everyday life, we need to live not only the first tone but the second as well. We feel best if we don't marginalize our overtones.

Our essence, our basic tendency or pilot wave, is the sum of all our sub-tones. The force of our dreaming is the sum of the way we normally live (approximated by the first fundamental tone) plus our deeper dreaming states. When all facets of these two states are combined, we feel like we are on the "right path," the path with heart.

By marginalizing our deepest states, we "collapse" our pilot waves into our most probable personalities, those dominant chunks of energy we identify as ourselves (see figure 8-4).

Our inner and outer worlds in dreamland are wavelike and coexist as spaces and hyperspaces, so weird things can happen. For example, one night you might dream that you are alive, sitting in a coffee shop, and then in the next dream fragment the same night, you may be dead. In a way, you are a sum of being both dead and alive. Your path with heart is the sum of being dead and alive. However, if you marginalize the sense of being dead in everyday reality, you will probably be bothered by fatigue and feel "dead." Instead you could be "dead" in the sense of being detached from your ordinary self in everyday life.

In any case, being both dead and alive at the same time can be your path with heart on that day. I recall Patanjali, the mythical parent of yoga, suggesting many centuries ago in India that the goal of yoga was to be a dead person in life.[6]

Parallel Worlds and the Path of the Heart

Hugh Everett[7] used the many-worlds paradigm in physics in the late 1950s by reinterpreting Schrödinger's wave equation. Everett said that those waves were the sums of other waves, separate states, which were "worlds"—that is, parallel worlds. He meant that each time we view an object (in consensus reality), we enter with it into one of its many possible states. The other states are still there. Similarly, other worlds are present, but we do not see them because they are parallel and do not intersect appreciably with the world in which we are standing at that given moment of observation.

Radical as this interpretation was, and still is, the many-worlds theory was accepted, in part, because leading physicists such as Richard Feynman, Murray Gell-Mann, and Stephen Weinberg agreed with the approach. Each separate quantum state of a system is a potential parallel world.

Loosely speaking, a "world" is a process, or a set of interacting processes, which essentially do not interfere with other processes in the superposition—that is, those processes that compose the general wave. To use an example from earlier in the text, being alive is one world; being dead is another, parallel world. Both worlds exist simultaneously. Sometimes worlds are referred to in physics as universes.

As noted, the psychological analogy to parallel worlds is the array of dream images and moods you have. You dream in any one night that you are alive, and then later, that you are dead. These two "worlds" are relatively separate. When you were in the dream of being alive, you were not aware of the dream of being dead. In addition, the world in which you saw yourself dead was more or less separate from the world of the first dream. When you awaken, your overall mood or state or universe is a combination (or a figurative superposition) of these various worlds.

Just as any state of mind (or state of a piece of matter) can be considered to be a summation of many states, the "universe" too can be considered to be composed of "all that can exist," as stated by Michio Kaku.[8] Likewise, all the various possible states of an object or person are present at any given instant, though the one we observe depends upon a summation that is weighted according to which is most likely at that moment.

Cosmologist Stephen Hawking took a great quantum leap in thinking about the world and the universe. He considered that the universe is also an object and suggested it is a quantum object.[9] Instead of applying quantum mechanics only to little particles, he assumed that quantum mechanics could be applied to the largest "particle"—the whole universe.

In trying to understand what happened at the moment of the universe's birth, Hawking proposed that the universe's pilot wave, like any other pilot wave, was the sum of many other waves—that is, other worlds or universes. Just as I pointed out in the earlier diagram (see figure 8-2) in this chapter, in the next diagram (see figure 8-5), the universe's wave is the sum of many other universes whose effects on the overall wave are suggested by the little bumps or hills.

The big bump on the left represents the universe we live in, the one physicists consider the most probable. However, the smaller hills to the right are other possible wave functions or universes.

While these ideas of Hawking are being debated in the science community, let me suggest that this way of thinking is very close to symbolic thinking in process-oriented psychology.

Each of us is a kind of universe with many relatively independent sub-universes. In one universe you may be an Islamic Afghan; while in another you are a European Christian or Jew; in another you are an Aboriginal Australian. Still in other universes you might be a bird flying freely in the air. Each of these universes contributes to the total sense you have of life.

In the next chapter, I discuss how Aboriginal peoples of Australia used an idea of parallel worlds called songlines centuries

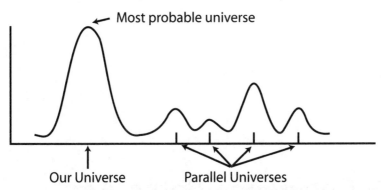

Figure 8-5. Wave Function of the Universe. Adapted from a drawing on the website of Michio Kaku and his discussions in his book *Hyperspace* (see www.mkaku.org).

before physics ever thought of such a concept. The concept of a quantum pilot wave underlying an object or the entire universe is a new version of the subtle feelings and inner sentient knowing that these peoples have used to guide them in their everyday lives.

According to Aboriginal beliefs, because the world was created by song, we can find our path through an unknown area by sensing its songs. Likewise, songlines can lead us through difficult areas of life. When out of touch with ourselves, loved ones, or our community, we can do as our ancestors did—and use songs, tones, and overtones to reestablish our sense of balance.

All these songs together—all the sounds of the moment—are guides through life. Remember to sense the sound within you, do it again right now (as explained earlier in the exercise), and then raise it by one octave. Finally, put the first sound and its overtone together, and you will experience a more magical way to connect to your world. Try it now; find the path with heart. That path is the momentary map of moving through the world you live in.

9 Coherence Baths As Quantum Medicine

If one looks deep within oneself there are not
only two worlds, there are so many worlds that it
is beyond expression. It can be understood that
one person lives only in the external world, while
another lives in two worlds, and a third person
may live in many worlds at the same time. . . .
When one asks, "Where are those worlds? Are
they above the sky or down below the earth?"
the answer is, "All worlds are in the same place
as we are."

—*Inayat Khan, a Sufi mystic who lived
in India and Persia in the early 1900s*[1]

According to a recent article in *Scientific American*, overtones play a significant role in the lives of many people today.[2]
Overtone singing is a form of vocal expression that has been
around as long as humans. Still today, peoples of the Middle East,

Western Asia, Tibet, Mongolia, Siberia, as well as the first peoples of South and North America, use overtone singing for healing purposes.

According to both scientific findings and Aboriginal spirituality, songlines rule the universe. The power of sound in Australian Aboriginal mythology is based upon the mythic figures that were believed to have created the Earth's formations in the Dreamtime, bringing natural species into life, creating cultures, customs, and rules. According to Bruce Chatwin, these mythic figures "wrapped the whole world in a web of song." In his book, *The Songlines,* he explains: "The land first exists as a concept in the mind and is given form through the singing."

We could also say that the body, as part of the land, in the larger sense, also has songlines. In fact, according to Aboriginal Australians, the vibratory song of an object must be known and sung before it can come alive. Not only objects, but also whole landscapes are organized by songlines. These nonconsensual songline pathways (called Yiri in the Walpiri language) cross the Earth and were created by mythical Aboriginal ancestors. As they rose out of the dark earth, these beings created "mountains, valleys, waterholes—and so singing, the world came into existence."[3]

To communicate with one another, distant groups of Aborigines used songlines or dreaming tracks. Aboriginal peoples believe that the real world exists only when they can both see and sing it. In fact, the Aboriginal word for "country" means "line." Both the object or the land *and* its songline create its reality.

Songlines are a kind of formula or law of life. While modern physics expresses such laws in terms of math, the Aboriginal peoples express laws as sounds, stories, and paintings.[4] In the painting which follows (Aboriginal art of Lorna Inkamana), you see a kind of quantum wave field of an area. Notice the snake that is considered to be the guardian of the Earth. Songlines depict the vibrations of life, the piloting information carried by the quantum waves of universe that lie "behind" our whole existence.

My experience of the Australian aboriginal people gives me a sense that the songs of a given group describe the pilot waves not

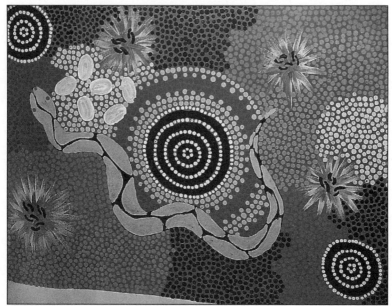

Figure 9-1. Snake Dreaming. This is a picture by Lorna Inkamana. Around the outstation where Lorna lives are the sites of numerous snake-dreaming stories. The snakes guard the waterholes to ensure that they are not befouled in any way.[5]

only of the Earth we live on but of organizations, cities, and communities—the deep and colorful realities connected with the sense of "home" and understanding of one another.

Realizing the potential physical and psychological effects of music, Aboriginal Australians listened to and "bathed in" sound, creating what particular individuals told me was called a "didgeridoo bath." In this ritual, the healer "blows" sounds and vibrations from a musical instrument called a didgeridoo into the body to create wellness.

In the last chapter, while learning to listen to the sounds, tones, and overtones in your body, you may have noticed a sense of wellness linked to your music. When immersed in fields of your own vibrations, you are "at home." You may have discovered how increased awareness or lucidity makes you feel more coherent, more connected with some larger path. Songlines, or pilots waves, can be experienced in your body's overtones.

Exercise: Healing Effects of Overtones—Overtone Symptom Work

Usually without realizing it, both the modern healer or doctor and her patient live in a sea of wonder, in a field of dreams under the influence of the force of silence. Let's explore this field in the following exercise that may reveal the sounds, "laws," and virtual patterns and worlds embedded in symptoms.[6]

Choose a symptom. When you are ready, think about the body symptoms you have now or have had in the past. Choose a particular chronic body symptom that you would like to focus on. If you have more than one, choose the symptom most troublesome to you. If you have no particular symptom in the moment, remember one you have had; this may be a symptom you have already worked on.

Focus on and feel that symptom. Feel or remember feeling it, and describe that feeling to yourself or to someone who is helping you. (One reader chose to focus on the feeling of a migraine headache.)

Make movements with your hands that represent that body feeling. When you sense you are expressing some aspect of that symptom, sing a tone out loud that corresponds to that particular body motion. Be patient, you may have to make several motions and sounds to find the right ones.

Feel your way into the parallel world of that sound and motion. This means, notice feelings and images and ideas that arise in connection with that sound and movement, trust them, and let them lead you in a fantasy in which that sound and motion play a role. The fantasy can be any length.

Explore shape-shifting. Bring out your playfulness—be a child or a shaman and climb into the world of that fantasy. Briefly explore how it feels to move about in that world until you sense its message. Remember or write down or tell your fantasy (your story) and your experience as you make the motion and sounds. Let your mind be creative, and write down your story as it unfolds. Let your imagination go. What is the story that came to you when you heard that tone? (The reader with the migraine headache made tapping motions with her hand and imagined a "bell" ringer who was awakening the people of her small town to new happenings.)

Make another sound, the overtone of the first tone. Do this by raising the first sound or tone by whatever you feel an octave might be. If it is too hard to raise the tone by an octave, go an octave lower. I first recommend you go up an octave, but if your voice cannot do that easily, go down an octave.

Let that overtone (or undertone) express itself. Make hand motions with the sound and catch the flickering images and ideas that come to you when you hear the overtone. Let a story unfold with the images of this tone. Don't work hard, just let a story quickly come to mind. What is that story? (For example, the person with the migraine heard a high-pitched alarm, telling her people of an emergency—an earthquake was about to occur. People should all move to a new area, to the safety of a mountain area where there were no quakes.)

Try to hear both tones at once, now that you have two tones and two stories. This can be a very creative moment. First try hearing both tones and stories at the same time. If you have a voice recorder, sing both sounds into it. Otherwise, you can sing the songs in your mind. Start by singing one tone, then the other tone, one after another.

Wait for your mind to allow these parallel worlds to connect. If you are patient and take the time, a coming together of the two tones and stories occurs spontaneously. Sometimes one song will dominate. Sometimes another. As you hear the first and the second, you might notice yourself creating an entirely new third sound, together with a resolving story. Wait for that to happen and express the resolution as a tale or sound. Ask yourself about the meaning of that story and sound.

This resulting experience can be very irrational and unexpected. Trust your movement and fantasy process, as the sounds and stories come together on their own. Be patient until this happens. (The bell ringer heard the higher-pitched alarm and made her message clear: It's time to leave for greater clarity and detachment. Following this experience, the woman left her job as a business advisor, and her migraine headaches left as well.)

Create a sound bath. Experiment recording the final sound, or combination of sounds, whatever it was. Record them and have a friend or your recorder play or "blow" the sound back to you or sing the song to the body part with the symptom. Tell yourself or your friend to "blow that sound toward the body part that has the symptom." If the whole body is involved, "bathe" all of it in the song. The idea is to create a vibrational world of meaning around your body, especially around the symptom area. When sound is played to—or "blown into"—your body, special sensations sometimes arise. Notice your experience. You may feel "thirsty" for that sound.

Repeat the sound bath. Blow that resolution back into the part of the body where the symptom is or was. Make the sound directly into the body area/part. Blow that vibe back to that body part and notice its effect on the symptom area.

Ask yourself: What have I discovered or learned about myself and my symptom by doing this exercise? Did you notice in what way your body symptom was a combination of parallel worlds, worlds you did not quite know about? Could you tell how the second sound was implied or embedded in the first? (Make the first sound, and try to hear the second "within" it.)

Carry the sound with you as you move about in your daily life. Whatever your experience, "bathe" and live in it until your body feels it is "understood." In doing so, you are "tuned in to," or on the same "wavelength" as your deepest self.

Write your story in your dream journal. It will help you understand the dreams you are having. Tell people your tale; perhaps it is part of your personal myth.

Ask yourself: How will I use these discoveries, my "songs," with myself in the near future? Can you imagine how they may influence or "move" you, for example, in your relationships, at work, or in the groups or communities of which you are part? (The person with headaches decided to become a "bell ringer" to those around her. Eventually, she became a significant political leader in her country.)

Describe what may have been "healing" through this experience. (The headache woman said what was healing was feeling that within her body problems lay a "vibration that transformed me into my real self.")

Your song and story convey hints about how to care for your body. You may have discovered one or more of the following points.

• Parallel worlds have different atmospheres, stories, and even "rules."

• Bringing awareness to parallel worlds gives your different parts a chance to know one another.

- Embedded within the fundamental tones of problem areas are overtone spaces that lead to resolutions.

- The tones and overtones of symptoms inadvertently resolve problems of everyday life that were not directly part of the symptom work.

- Body symptoms are pathological only from a CR perspective. From the viewpoint of dreamland, symptoms reflect the known world and new parallel worlds.

- From the viewpoint of dreamland, body symptoms are unsung songs. No body process is "wrong." Illness is simply a suitcase with unpacked musical gifts. Your symptoms are not just a part of an ill body but a group of parallel worlds waiting to be "sung."

Quantum State Crossover

Connecting to parallel worlds can relieve symptoms. Inversely, ignoring or belittling parallel world experiences leaves you feeling uneasy and irritates your body because you are ignoring a part of your path, a part of your guiding wave. If you are excited but act quiet, you feel nervous. If you are tired but act energetic, you become uneasy. Any nuance that is neglected is experienced as a symptom or part of a symptom. On the other hand, if you live with awareness and accept all your worlds, your body is relieved.

Research implies that not only people but also plants grow better when certain music is played to them. Peter Tompkins and Christopher Bird, in their *The Secret Life of Plants* (1989), describe how plants seemed to love the music of Schubert, Bach, and Beethoven, but when rock was played to them, they grew in the opposite direction, away from the radio. When the music of Ravi Shankar was played, plants grew horizontally toward the loudspeakers playing the music.

I call the experience of mind-body connection that occurs while hearing or feeling the sounds of symptoms "the quantum state crossover." An overlapping or crossover occurs between psychology and biology, between the psychological meaning of the sounds and the biophysics of your symptoms. This crossover occurs because of the unity of, or similarity between, the patterns found in both worlds. The crossover phenomenon points to the existence of some single world, the essence world behind the parallel experiences that occur on levels we currently label as psychology, physics, and medicine.

Aboriginal beliefs about sound coupled with your own experiences of overtones may give you a sense of what is meant by *subatomic body states* and the *biology of life.* Immeasurable quantum waves are analogous to the vibratory songlines that are the sounds and tunes, the songs and myths, that move us.

The Coherence of the Pilot Wave

The quantum state crossover hypothesis suggests a coherence—or even a one-to-one correspondence—between altered states of consciousness and the quantum sub-states of the pilot wave. The tones you make to describe your symptoms represent experiences that are not entirely measurable in modern consensus reality. These tones reveal your body's tendencies. I use the term "body tendency" synonymously with quantum wave tendency, but each is more appropriate in its own context. Thus, the body's subatomic states or quantum waves are the physicist's terms for what the therapist might call subpersonalities, overtones, or dream fragments.[7] In this way, the realms of physics, psychology and biology "cross over."

By ignoring or marginalizing our various tendencies, tones, and overtones, we get "out of synch" with ourselves, which we sense as dis-ease, un-easiness, lack of orientation, or depression. The opposite of marginalization is lucid awareness and tuning in to our various sub-states and following them. In everyday reality, resolving this sense of being out of synch with ourselves is called healing.

I would like to be more exact about the general meaning of healing. It refers to *coherence* among your awareness and the states you experience. *Coherence* refers to at least a short-term, one-to-one correspondence between elements in different systems which have identical or similar form, shape, or structure. This is called isomorphism. An analogy or similarity is isomorphic when what happens in one system happens in the other.

For example, if a city map is accurate, it is coherent with the city. Each point on the map corresponds to an analogous point in the city. If spots on the map, like Broadway and Main Street, do not correspond to those given points in the city in a point-to-point manner, you get lost; you are out of synch with that city.

I have suggested that our altered states of consciousness and our subatomic states are coherent. By doing the last exercise, I hope you experienced something about the coherence between your everyday map of life and your body: You feel best when your everyday mind is coherent and as diverse as the spectrum of images and sounds of your rainbow body.

You get confused about life—feel "lost"—if the "map" you are using is not coherent with the "territory" through which you are moving. In such times, use awareness to notice the map created by your body symptoms, to help yourself get in synch with your body and your life as a whole.

The map is an analogy of your awareness of your inner patterns. If the map you use to get along in the world ignores certain regions, those regions eventually reach your attention by rebelling. If your map is incomplete, your body lets you know. Try it. Whenever you feel uneasy, open your suitcase and unpack your map, that is, the tones and overtones of your body. Become more coherent. Bring those sounds into everyday life; make it richer and more interesting.

Then you may experience healing as a kind of bathing in a deep sense of knowing, in the waves that guide us. Remember that wisdom; those waves are imbedded in body symptoms. The sounds and overtones relieve symptoms by synchronizing us with the deepest self. I call this synchronization experience "the quantum state crossover." It bridges psychology and biology, the meaning of the sounds and the biophysics of your body.

II

NONLOCAL MEDICINE: THE WORLD IN SYMPTOMS

10 How Community Influences the Body

Einstein characterized the strangeness of this situation [being able to predict only probabilities and not actualities] . . . by referring to the wave function as a "ghost field."
—*Robert Nadeau and Menas Kafatos*[1]

To the everyday mind, we live and work alone or together with others in our communities. However, in the images of dreamland, we live in a kind of "ghost field," a web or mixture of real people and what I call "community ghosts" or projections in our organizations. To our dreaming mind, a so-called "organization" is not just a clustering of real people and buildings and issues; it is also an inextricable mixture of almost unimaginable spirits that care for, disrespect, teach, and spook one another.

From the essence viewpoint, the community made up of real people and dreamland ghosts, projections, and feelings is hardly imaginable, and indeed feels more like a power motivated by the force of silence. One possible dreamland version of this group essence's nature might be gleaned by imagining yourself as a fish swimming in the quantum sea of virtual waves that lies "behind" or "beneath" the CR reality of people and worlds. As a fish swimming around in this essence, your movements create waves around you, just as you are formed and moved by the waves of other fish in this sea. These waves form and "in-form" us all, just as every move we make is felt by fish everywhere.

In the first part of this book, we saw how the "sea"—the intentional field—expresses itself in tendencies toward certain directions. These tendencies, like the quantum waves which describe them theoretically, are a central intersecting point between psychology and physics. Unfolding these tendencies in terms of images and stories creates parallel worlds, hyperspaces, and a virtual spectrum of experience. In chapter 9, I introduced the idea of the quantum state crossover, based upon the similarity in form between the rhythmic sound experiences of altered states of consciousness and quantum waves. We saw how awareness of symptom vibrations makes us more coherent and has potential healing effects. In Rainbow Medicine, the body appears not only as a Newtonian mechanical object of flesh and bones, but as a rainbow, a spectrum of experiences described by sounds and tones. In the rainbow view, symptoms are not just problems, but *awareness indicators* pointing to parts of the spectrum wanting to be noticed.

In part 2, we will study nonlocal aspects of Rainbow Medicine by connecting the experience of symptoms to problems in relationships, community, and the world. My goal is to bring forward a basic principle: Nonlocal patterns seek realization by using the local nature of our bodies and relationships. By exploring the nonlocality of body experiences, you will feel how your community affects your body,[2] and also how your body experiences may resolve community problems.

Nonlocality in Biology

"Nonlocality" is a new term for an ancient idea. In chapter 9, I spoke of the Tuva people of northern Mongolia. In their belief system, a mountain is real not only because of its locality but also because of its nonlocality. Its locality is described by its shape and location, and its nonlocality is known in terms of its "voice"—the sound of the wind moving around the mountain. This voice has a quality of nonlocality because we can't say exactly where it is. Though a particular particle of air may have a location and time, the wind does not speak from a given point. The voice of the mountain is a dreamland or feeling concept.

Likewise, you are basically located in your physical body. But then, you may dream about something happening in the world around you and the next day it actually happens. The dream is like the wind in the forest; dreams are nonlocal aspects of your nature. You exist in both consensus reality and in nonconsensus reality. You are local and nonlocal. One of my friends woke up from a vivid dream of a winter storm in which waves crashed against a pier and destroyed most of it. When she got up the next morning, she heard on the news that a pier located about 25 miles from her home had been destroyed by a storm—which had barely visited her locale.

The multidimensionality of our biology and our world is one reason why we sometimes fail to solve body problems by solely addressing one body location. Local medicine ignores the nonlocal nature of the person and field in which the body lives. In Rainbow Medicine, symptom work is both local and nonlocal. You work on your body and, by touching the quantum and dream levels of experience, simultaneously work on your relationships and the whole world.

An interesting example of a living body connected to nonlocal fields is the homing pigeon. This bird is known to find its way home after having been locked up and carried hundreds of miles away. Research shows that neither smell nor the Earth's magnetic field nor memory can explain the homing pigeon's knowing where its home is. Dogs and other animals seem to possess similar abilities.

Such knowing prompted nonmechanistic currents of thought in biology, notably the work of Rupert Sheldrake, an English biologist

Pilot Waves and Morphogenetic Fields

Refer again to my diagram, Flight of an Electron (figure 7-1, p. 73) in chapter 7, about the wave-like behavior of a particle in area II, before it is observed.

In area II, the wave function or pilot wave is nonlocal, in the sense of being everywhere, until it is "collapsed" by measurement in area III. The guiding wave in area II is, according to the math of physics, everywhere in the universe. It is a "tendency" without specific location until we collapse it by becoming aware of tendencies and their meaning and movements in our bodies.

Though the wiggle in area II is drawn as if it were in between areas II and III, the wave function before detection is theoretically anywhere and everywhere in time and space. Only upon detection does it "collapse" (which can be restated as "marginalizing its nonlocal aspects").[3] Thus any physical object in nonconsensual or mathematical reality is everywhere in the universe.

who first came to public notice in 1981 with his *A New Science of Life: The Hypothesis of Formative Causation.* Sheldrake named the nonlocal aspect of our world—that which guides the pigeon home—the "morphogenetic field." This nonconsensual, immeasurable field has many qualities that remind me of quantum mechanics and especially of Bohm's idea of virtual pilot waves.[4]

Nonlocality is considered a central feature of modern physics. Quantum theory involves nonlocal connection between particles separated in space and time. This theory has been confirmed experimentally so many times that, in spite of early objections from physicists such as Einstein, science today accepts as fact that particles from the same source remain connected as if the spatial and temporal distance between them did not exist.[5]

Two particles, such as photons of light from the same light bulb or source, remain linked over hundreds of years and thousands of miles. If something happens to one particle, the other "knows it." This connection is due to the "notorious" behavior of the pilot wave which evolves not in consensus reality's time and space but in the multidimensional mathematical spaces described by physicists.

The wave is like a dream. Think of a dream of yourself and another person. That dream is anywhere in the night you dream it. During the day, it often proves true that you and the other person are somehow connected.

The philosopher Robert Nadeau and physicist Menas Kafatos discuss nonlocality in terms of particles such as photons of light (coming from a single source) and make the "dramatic conclusion that nonlocality is a fundamental property of the entire universe." They go further: "The foundation of physical reality is actually 'nonlocal,'" a discovery the authors view as "the most momentous in the history of science."[6]

Thus the quantum wave of an object, and our dreamland experience of guiding waves in the form of the intentional fields, are everywhere in the universe, even though they are most intensely experienced around their respective objects and people. Likewise, songlines are felt inside us but, at the same time, spread out in the world, indeed, in the whole universe. In dreaming, we are in dreamland, moving freely, wherever our tendencies lead us.

Nonlocality in Groups

Magicians and sorcerers have always tried to tap into the underlying reality of nonlocality to heal or trouble others from a distance. Voodoo is perhaps the most widely known of these practices. This practice depends, in part, upon spirits that can possess the healer as well as move anywhere they are needed.

Though most of us would not identify ourselves, when in a group setting, as involved in some form of witchcraft or healing ritual, at one time or another we may have experienced a nonlocal element in relationships and community. At one time or another, you may not have been able to "get someone out of [your] mind" and felt possessed by thoughts of this person. Therapists usually localize such thoughts by calling them projections. However, there is a nonlocal aspect to all of these thoughts. Nonlocal elements—in this context, projections and feelings about others—are the very core of what we experience as interconnectedness and community.

Nonlocality

When I use the term *nonlocality* to refer to a timeless and "spaceless" connection between people and parts, I mean:

• *The interactions between us do not diminish with space.* When particles such as photons come from the same source, they remain linked with one another, regardless of distance and time.[7] Distance does not influence connection (except to the degree that we erect CR beliefs about the effects of distance on connection, which then influence our perception of dreamland events). Likewise, in psychology, if we were once close to a certain person, even many years ago, we are always connected, regardless of where we live today or how long it has been since we had any form of contact. If you love (or dislike) someone, you are connected to

that person, regardless of how far away she or he lives.

• *The interactions between us are not bound by the limitations of the speed of light.* Einstein said that things on this Earth could not go faster than the speed of light. That means that when we communicate with voice, e-mail, or telephone, our signals cannot go faster than the speed of light. However, nonlocal interactions make communication appear as if it can go so fast that it can even go backward in time. In the time-like spaces of dreamland, what you do in the future influences you—and me—today.

• *The interactions between us can go from here to there without going through the intervening space.* We cannot track the path of our communication exactly in space or in time.

Process-oriented group work, or "worldwork," addresses consensual aspects of groups, such as issues, facts, and problems. To have a lasting effect on groups, worldwork addresses the nonconsensual atmosphere or community "field," noticing how that field expresses itself in terms of "timespirits"—that is, those specific and typical roles that slowly change over time.[8]

Experience with many thousands of people worldwide has shown me that applying related worldwork techniques influences organizational and city-level fields.[9] Part of the rationale for using dreamlike techniques and role-play is that such roles, like every-thing in dreamland, are nonlocal. For example, the typical "good" and "bad" roles, such as the persecutor and the persecuted, can be found in just about everyone, everywhere, at one time or another.

Thus the atmosphere of a group exists beyond the local boundaries of a given community's location; indeed, the "dream-ing" of the community is everywhere. Any time you think of a nation or group located at such-and-such a spot on the planet, you connect to the nonlocal intentional wave, or the force of silence, of that community, which is everywhere. Thus, in a way, any war is a world war, any conflict is world conflict. That is why most wars are never resolved in one area alone. They can only be repressed in a given locality. For resolutions to last, everyone everywhere must resolve war.

We human beings, as well as all the particles in the universe, are entangled and coupled through nonlocal connections. From the context of Rainbow Medicine, health and illness are consen-sual events in time and space requiring nonlocal awareness work.

The Group's Force of Silence

Psychology has long dealt with one-to-one human experi-ences and relationships. The governing paradigm is that people are conscious and unconscious, real and dreaming. In my way of thinking, groups are similar. They are full of real people and objects, but they also are a "community" because of the nonlocal roles and essence feelings. When a community is coherent with its dreaming, it is "at home" with the songs of the land and the behav-ior of each member.

Communication in groups occurs in various worlds simultane-ously, as follows:

I. Causal Communication of CR Groups: You and I connect when we shake hands; we communicate through physical con-tact. We connect through the viruses that we share; I sneeze, and you breathe it in. We connect through the telephone, e-mail (and its viruses *there*, too!), radio, TV, through friends, and so on.

II. Dreamland or Hyperspatial Communication: We connect through dreams and through our collective visions and hopes. We communicate in dreamland through projections and the subtle feelings we have about one another. If you or *I alone* change, we may *both* feel different, even if there has been no consensual communication between us. We share dream figures, roles, ghost roles, and so on. Dreamland connections are nonlocal; we are all entangled.

III. Essence Level Communication: In everyday life, we are different from one another. In dreamland, we are both different and the same. However, at the essence level, we are indistinguishable from one another. At this level we only sense a force of silence that includes everything and everyone.

The essence of a community has many names—*Earth, home, love, common ground, the Great Spirit, God,* to name a few. The essence of a community, its intentional field, is everywhere within and beyond a particular location in space or time. Thus, in a way, we can kill a group of people, but we cannot kill their intentional field since it is an immortal spirit which appears repeatedly. (Aboriginal Australians say we can kill the kangaroo but not the kangaroo dreaming.)

In those rare moments when we are aware of a community's force of silence, we sense ourselves as different faces of some Great Spirit, and we can validate both our differentness and our sameness.[10] I remember an Aboriginal elder from Adelaide, Uncle Lewis (also known as Mr. Lewis O'Brien), who showed me how the whole city of Adelaide was organized according to a force of silence he referred to as "the Red Kangaroo."[11] He discovered that the street map of Adelaide turned out to be an image of the Red Kangaroo.

The basic idea is that the kangaroo is an expression representing the force of silence of that town. In general, a community is a combination of its CR facts, the images of dreamland, and the force of silence behind it. Further, all events, including our momentary experiences in that area, are organized by the silent force of its dreaming.

Exercise: How Group Atmosphere Creates Body Music That Influences Symptoms

To explore the interconnection between yourself and your community:

Take a few breaths, when you are ready, and make yourself comfortable. Think about a group or community that you are part of and would like to understand better. (Alternatively, you can also think of a family, city, or national situation.)

Is that group located in a given area or spread throughout the world? Think about that community, wherever its members are located, and recall the kinds of issues or tensions it is dealing with. How would you designate one of its issues?

Now let's explore how that community connects with your body. Group Sound: Pretend that your community or family is in the midst of working on the issue you just recalled. For example, your group may be working on relationship problems between members, economic problems, or discussing matters of creativity or spirituality.

Feel the atmosphere of the group by imagining people interacting on that issue. What do you imagine the people are doing? What does the situation look like? What does it feel like? Use both hands to express the situation symbolically. What are your hands and arms doing?

When you are ready, make a sound that represents the atmosphere of the group in the midst of working on its topic. Make a note of this sound or record it. Let's call this the "group sound." For example, one reader focused on the conflict between two smaller subgroups in her community. The atmosphere was tense and threatening. To express this atmosphere in sound—to represent the terror and the terrorizing actions happening between the members of the subgroups in conflict—the reader shrieked.

Body Symptom Sounds. Now let's explore how the situation affects your body. How does the atmosphere around that topic make you feel physically? Imagine the topic again, imagine people discussing things, feel the atmosphere, and feel what it is like to be in that atmosphere. Notice how that atmosphere affects your body. Imagine a given moment: Are you quiet? Are you tense, nervous, afraid, angry, detached? (My reader felt terrified and angry.)

What does this atmosphere do to one of your chronic symptoms? Choose a symptom and feel what the atmosphere does to that symptom. (Sometimes breathing into the symptom can heighten your feeling and focus on it.) If you have no chronic symptoms, just focus on your overall body state. If possible, however, sense one of your chronic symptoms, even if it is mild (e.g., a slightly lifted shoulder, tilted neck, shallow breathing, and so on). Check out what the atmosphere does to that symptom. How is the symptom exaggerated or relieved by the atmosphere? For example, do you feel itchy, burning, or trembling? Pounding pressure? One of my readers, whose symptom was high blood pressure, now felt a pounding sensation in her chest.

Now let a sound emerge that represents the experience of how your chronic symptom is affected by the atmosphere. For example, my reader with the high blood pressure said she experienced the pounding sound of drums in her chest area.

Now let a story come to mind around this rhythm and sound. For example, my reader connected the drums with warriors going on the warpath and being killed in battle.

When you are ready, make a second sound an octave higher (or lower, if that is easier) and catch the fantasy image and story from that sound. This is your overtone experience. For example, raising the drumming sound an octave higher released a fantasy from that reader of herself as a child beating drums, having a great time, playing and enjoying herself.

Bring your overtone and its story together with the sound representing the way your chronic symptom is affected by the group. Let your creativity connect the overtone sound and story with the chronic symptom tone and its story. An easy way to do this is to hear the chronic symptom sound and story and its overtone's sound and story, and be a witness to the new sound(s). Just let the sounds and stories connect. You may notice how one sound leads, then another, or how a third sound emerges as the sounds come together. Take your time with this part.

Notice the fantasy that emerges from this new experience and how it affects your body and your symptom. For example, when the playfulness of the child entered the reader's heart, she became more playful and wanted to play with everyone , instead of fighting against them. Her imagined blood pressure symptom felt better, and she imagined how she could "play" with her group.

Let's call this last sound your "resolving sound." Record it and how it affects your symptom. Now let's work on bringing the resolving sound to your group or world.

Concluding Sound. To bring your *resolving body symptom sound* together with the *group sound* that you recorded in the beginning of this exercise, remember them both. Then make one sound then the other. Notice the first, then the second and the resulting experience. Do the sounds tend to follow one another? Does just one or the other sound finally remain? Or a totally new song and sound emerge? Keep your attention on what is happening until a concluding sound emerges.

When you "have" your concluding sound, let a story about that sound unfold. What is happening in this final sound and story? How did they come about? Think about how this concluding sound and story might occur in reality. How is that story already occurring in some subtle way?

For example, the group's "shrieking" sound came together with the child's playful drumming, and a new sound-song emerged which was a kind of shrieking with fun. A fantasy emerged in which she acted out the conflicting roles in the group as if they were two dolls talking to one another!

The woman who did this exercise said that her playfulness had already been happening in a subtle way. Until now, every time she thought of her group, she not only got the feelings of high blood pressure, but at the same time had to giggle about something, without knowing why. In any case, at their next meeting, the woman did just what she experienced in this exercise; she played out the arguing parties herself, using both her hands as if they were two puppets, talking to one another. Everyone laughed.

Make a note about this subtle occurrence for the future. If you are in a creative mood and have a moment more, make a sketch of some comic-book or fairy-tale figure, a puppet, or spontaneous person-like image of someone who might represent the essence of your concluding sound and story.

Thinking about This Experiment

There are many ways to think about what happened in this exercise. In a Rainbow Medicine view, the group sound represents only one of its dreamland songlines—that is, a particular altered state or sub-state of your community. Your body experiences (and those of other people) are other sub-states of that community. Usually, a group runs into trouble because it chooses some sub-states and people to focus on but marginalizes other states of consciousness and the individuals who represent these states. The total sum of all the sub-states is the community process, its pilot wave, just as your force of silence and intentional wave are the sum of all your separate feelings, dream figures, and/or sub-states.

Such a general sum might be diagrammed as follows:

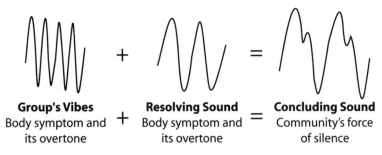

Group's Vibes		**Resolving Sound**		**Concluding Sound**
Body symptom and	**+**	Body symptom and	**=**	Community's force
its overtone		its overtone		of silence

Figure 10-1. Community Essence or Force of Silence

The concluding sound and feeling are connected to the community's core, its deepest essence. This core is its greatest power, the community's force of silence.

In the terms of the preceding exercise, the essence is experienced as the "concluding sound," the force of the community's dreaming. This sound and force, though usually unconscious, are a rallying point for the whole community, something everyone will be able to relate to, even though in a given moment the essence may be forgotten amidst the focus on a given CR situation. That force is always there in the background, creating the diversity of situations and the various viewpoints and aspects of the organization. In principle, the community's essence is the common ground shared by all of its members.

Your various body experiences and your different aspects are part of the community's CR and nonconsensus realities; likewise, the group and its conflicts are parts of you. The group affects your body, just as your awareness work and coherence with your "self" and community can help solve the community's problems. Your deepest feelings not only change you, yourself, but also the dreaming/feeling situation of the group . . . even *before* you interact with them in CR. In retrospect, it sometimes seems as if our community essences use "our" body symptoms as antennae for attracting resolutions to the community's problems.

Other Ways of Using Sound

There are many ways you can use sound to resolve community or one-to-one relationship problems and feel better. For example, during a tense conversation in relationship to someone, feel the atmosphere between the two of you. Is it tense or troubled? Feel the effect it has on your body, and make sounds and overtones as in the above exercise. With practice, you can do this rapidly to find the force of silence, the basic path which is the sum of these sounds. This is the path through difficult relationship terrain, the map of the territory.

Similarly, during a group process, feel the atmosphere, feel your body symptoms and their overtones, and bring your sounds and song (or their verbal significance) directly to your community. For example, in one of my Portland classes, a group process arose around the issues of love, heterosexism, and the marginalization of gays. Some people spoke against gay and lesbian relationships, while another group spoke on behalf of gays. At one point, the story of a gay teenager was told. Apparently the teen wanted to commit suicide because of the agony of living in a world where she was not wanted.

The tension in the room between the opposing groups was difficult on everyone. Suddenly, one courageous woman came forward, crying. She said she heard sounds within herself during the tense group process. Instead of speaking about those sounds, she sang the following song for that gay teenager.

"Don't worry; try not to turn onto problems which upset you.
Oh, don't you know, everything's all right,
we want you to sleep well tonight."

These words were inspired by the play *Jesus Christ Superstar.* As she sang, everyone felt the compassion the song conveyed for that teenager, and everyone fell silent. The song offered a common ground: It spoke to Christian fundamentalists by referring to Jesus, while simultaneously identifying the teenager as Christ.

When you experience such special moments in groups, you know that scientific thinking about nonlocality is insufficient to explain how the power or force of a community's dreaming influences us as individuals. However, you might also think as I do, that the patterns of physics and psychology are helpful in understanding exactly what Einstein meant when he called the quantum wave patterns "ghost fields."

11 Relationship Trouble Is Hyperspatial Medicine

Lovers don't finally meet, they are in each other all along.

—*Rumi*

Just as the nonlocal atmosphere of a CR group makes it a community, the dreaming of a person makes her a human being. In dreamland, anyone and everyone belongs to the community merely by thinking of it. Everything that is part of dreaming, including its roles and ghosts, is part of the "community," though these things may not be part of the CR group. Likewise, in dreamland you, as an individual, are everyone and everything you have ever thought of, as well as everyone who thinks about you.

It seems almost obvious that good friends improve your dream landscape and make you feel well. However, in this chapter, you will discover that enemies also have healing potential—in fact, they may be your most potent body medicine.

117

Atmospheres and Auras

The dreamland aspect of individuals and relationships consists, in part, of immeasurable atmospheres, feelings, fields, or auras around the people involved. This atmosphere is what gives us a nonlocal link—that is, a sense of connectedness. At one time or another, you have probably felt that couples, families, and perhaps even particular groups exude a kind of aura around them. Auras can feel thick, light, heavy, sticky, ecstatic, or even seem to stink.

Anyone who thinks about a couple takes part in their dreaming and is part of their relationship field. Thus, third parties, ex-partners, chairs, desks, apartments, children, parents, grandparents—all are part of the dreamland of your relationship. They are roles in your relationship's field at a given moment.

The nonlocal nature of atmospheres and auras makes the interconnections *spaceless;* that is, some events between people and parts are connected by signals that seem to go faster than the speed of light. Connections occur as if by magic. In relationships, you can move from where you are to where the other person is without crossing any in-between spaces. Further, your pasts and futures are contained in that atmosphere as well. Fields around bodies are typical auric emanations. In figure 11-1, you see a modern and a medieval depiction of this.

Nonlocal Mythic Principles

Nonlocal connections are typical of psychological and biological systems. Many people will say they feel better when someone they love sends them love. There is mounting evidence that if someone prays for you, you recuperate more quickly from an illness.[1]

Are there governing laws between human systems? As an individual, you may sense that your general pattern or personal myth seems to somehow bind past and present events so that they seem to fit in to who you are. Whatever happens, you follow

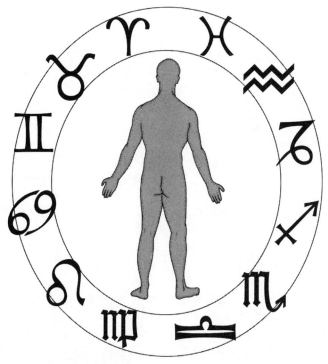

Figure 11-1. Sketches of Fields around the Body. In the picture above,[2] medieval Europeans made connections between the body, herbs, minerals, times of the year, and the planets. This picture shows some kind of coherence between the people and their world, for it depicts a universal law governing the body and connecting it to the rest of the universe. There is entanglement or interconnectedness between the parts of the universe and the human body. Our experiences are informed by the same dreamland or quantum information available to the rest of the world.

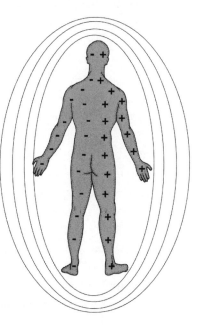

What Is Entanglement?

The phenomenon of entanglement that typifies quantum systems occurs due to some overarching laws. For example, in the quantum world, the sum of the spins (a type of quantized angular momentum) of a system's parts (such as its particles) must remain the same.

According to another basic law of physics, energy in an enclosed system must remain essentially constant. This balance in the energy is what makes things entangled, so that something's energy increases only if something else goes down. In nonlocal systems, where there are no visible spatial connections, general energy (conservation) laws govern everything that happens. Such overarching laws entangle the system's parts, which means that the parts are interdependent; they are entangled or tied together, for example by the requirement that the overall energy remain about the same.

Thus the parts are no longer entirely separable. According to physics, the elementary constituents of all matter are entangled because of natural laws. Entangled parts are like people in two parts of a room connected by (invisible) strings. What one person does is entangled with what the other does!

your pattern, however you define that. Some people are always running from something, others always turn into heroines and fight dragons, and so on. Minor changes in this pattern occur, but by and large, the basic configuration of the pattern remains the same.

In a way, your personal story, your myth, is a governing law. This means that whatever happens must be entangled or interconnected with everything else about you by the law of your life's pattern. Likewise, your body experiences and relationships are entangled not only with your own personal myth but those of others. The patterns of the force of silence expressed in auras and atmospheres entangle us all. We are beings entangled not only by the conservation of energy but also by a dreaming power that unfolds as the story of our lives and communities.

Nonlocal Body Connections

Jung called nonlocal connections between people and events "synchronicity," by which he meant "acausal orderedness." These noncausal connections occur as a result of their shared "meaning," the word Richard Wilhelm used for the Tao.[3] Two events would constitute a synchronicity, according to Jung, if they had the same meaning, or using Wilhelm's term, the same Tao.

Because the force of silence—your pilot wave—is a nonlocal potential source of information, all your sub-states and fantasies, aches and pains, and relationship problems are entangled with the whole world. In principle then, every illness is an "environmental illness" in the sense of being influenced by, and influencing, the world.

Usually the term "environmental illness" is used to refer to CR-based toxins and allergens that affect our bodies.[4] In what follows, however, we explore a more general kind of environmental illness connected with the atmosphere of relationships.

Phrases such as "he (or she) is a pain in the neck" or "a pain in the rear end" show our sense of the nonlocal connections between our bodies and our relationships. Because others disturb your body, working on relationships should (theoretically) help with your symptoms. The others you fantasize about out there are in your body as well.

Exercise: The Hyperspace of a Troublesome Person

In the following exercise, I ask you to focus on your body and the feelings you have about certain people. To profit the most from this training exercise, have a pencil and paper at hand.

Body Question: Settle yourself in a comfortable position and notice your breathing for a couple of minutes. While you are focusing on your breathing, ask yourself a question that has been puzzling you about your body. You might ask how you can solve some particular body symptom or what its meaning is. Make a note of this question because we will come back to it later.

Relationships: When you are ready, think about a person who has been troubling you either recently or in the past. Think of the most troublesome person you can imagine. What is that person like? Are they strong, nasty, loud, quiet, obsequious, etc.? Make a note of your descriptions.

Energy Field: While thinking of that person, imagine the field around her or him. What is the atmosphere, the space, or the aura like around that person? Use your imagination to picture the motions, colors, and forms near or around that person. For example, is her or his field full of darts, or dark clouds, or red splashes of water? Take a moment and actually draw this aura. What you draw may or may not be surprising to you.

Looking at your picture, ask yourself: Which of the colors or motions in the picture—which energy—is most difficult for me? For example, his piercing motions, dark red spots, or swirling emptiness may be the most disturbing for you.

How is this energy nonlocal for you? That is, in what way do you sense this energy in other situations in your life, in other people or events? Is this energy popping up now? Has it appeared at other times in other areas of your life? For example, do you find it in your work? Do other people with this energy generally upset you? It may be challenging to think about because we usually repress difficult energies.

Energy in Body: Use your hands and draw that difficult energy in the air. While moving your hands, sense your body and guess where that most difficult energy might be located. Draw a simple sketch of your body and mark the location of that energy. (There may be more than one location.) Do you currently have, or have you had, aches and pains or fears of illness there?

Essence of the Energy: Now we are going into the essence, the root of this field. To do this, act out the energy that is most difficult for you. Let it move your hands, or your whole body if you prefer. Use your awareness; don't move in a way that will injure yourself. Rather, become a shaman and carefully let go of your form as a human being; shape-shift, moving into and becoming this troublesome energy. Dance it or use your hands to express it.

When you are ready, ask yourself: What is the basic tendency of this energy? What was this energy in its earliest stage, before it got so big? To find the essence, it is sometimes helpful to make the motion more slowly while feeling the same intensity of the motion. (For example, a dart-like motion might become concentrated focus upon one thing at a time.)

If you still resist this basic tendency of that energy, go deeper. You have not yet arrived at its essence. There is no duality at the essence level. Go deeper and get to the essence of this troublesome energy. For example, the essence may finally appear to be a kind of sensitivity, or a flower, rock, spark of life, a quieting motion, clarity, or a mindlessness of some sort. Make a note of it.

Allow yourself to move into and live, for the moment, in this hyperspace, in the essence of that troublesome energy. What is its world like? Explore this space. Make up a story about it. What do you see there, feel there, and hear there?

Imagine some real or mythic figure, a human-like figure that represents this space, and become that figure now. Do you see yourself as a wise old rock-like woman, a giant bird, or a human-like feather in the wind? A young child in a cave?

Bring this essence into your everyday reality: How might this essence influence your lifestyle as a whole? How might this essence influence the way you relate to others? How might this essence influence your symptom area? Where might the essence figure be located in your body? Can you feel it there? Experience the figure there, relate to it there, *be* it.

Imagine using this figure in relationship with that original troublesome person. Perhaps you can be this essence figure with that person. Imagine how the difficult person would react. If you could bring that figure/essence out into the world, into the universe, how would it interact with and change the world?

Relate these experiences back to answer your original question about your body in the first step of this exercise. Do these experiences somehow answer that question?

Consider the possibility that the essence figure personifies the hyperspaces around you, an aspect of the pilot wave in the background of your life. Notice how the various experiences of your life are entangled in such a way as to bring this experience to your conscious awareness.

Many people who have tried this exercise discovered that their essence figure helped them to relate to the troublesome person in a very different and less stressful way. Some gained a totally different perspective on relationships as well as on their bodies.

I asked one of my students to write out an example of this exercise. Here is what she said:

"A particular man was bothering me some months back. This person is not a great character. I know that this troublesome person is somehow me, but as a whole, I do not feel the way he does! I just can't stand him!

"When I think about this man, I realize, he radiates a sort of dark cloud around him that makes others dislike him as well. In any case, that sort of energy upsets me. He always wants me to do something extra, just for him! Worse, if I don't, he gets terribly upset. And he acts depressed and produces a big dark cloud until I do something for him. Ugh! If he were not in my group of friends, I would never have anything to do with him.

"In any case, your exercise got me to thinking about how I create such clouds as well. I could not quite get how *all that* is me, but I surely felt where that dark cloud is in my body! Every time I lift something, I hurt my shoulder—there is a sort of spasm, a cramp, a heavy cloud of weight cramps up there! I know I should not lift things that hurt my shoulder, but it seems as if I can never learn!

"When I followed the steps of your training exercise, I found the essence of that energy, of that person's nonlocal relationship field. The essence of his darkness was a mysteriousness and an awesome unknowingness that fogs me over so that I no longer know where I want to go. That essence forces me to just give in to where 'it' wants to go. That nasty guy and my shoulder problem bother me so much to show me something mysterious and awesome that wants to move me along in life. A new way to live. Hosting this unknowingness not only helped my shoulder but also totally changed my relationship with that person. I even found myself being thankful for the way he is!"

The Force of Silence behind Relationships Is Medicine

In general, relationships get stuck because you see your enemies not as marginalized parts of yourself, of your intentional field, but as real people only. Perhaps your problem in relationships is seeing only one world, the CR world, and marginalizing the others. In this CR-only world, you see yourself as a person separate from all other persons. Marginalization and xenophobia make *you* and the *other* into separate human beings. In parallel worlds, in contrast, you and your friends are not discrete people but an unknown *shared* field of intensity, a force creating you and others.

The basic paradigm behind nonlocal relationship and community work is best summed up by Rumi's statement quoted at the beginning of this chapter. "Lovers don't finally meet, they are in each other all along." I would like to add the two words, "enemies and" to Rumi's beautiful statement which now becomes: "Enemies and lovers don't finally meet, they are in each other all along."

In other words, relationship trouble mirrors the spaces you share with others. Turbulent relationship and group problems reflect marginalization of those shared, nonlocal spaces and influence your CR body. By noticing the way in which relationship problems touch or in-form your body, you become aware of sounds and fields, aspects of yourself and the world around you which you have ignored or denied. By experiencing the common ground, the essence of these fields resolves body and relationship problems and restores a basic feeling of wellness. By pointing to symptoms and neglected dimensions of your rainbow body, relationship trouble is hyperspatial medicine.

By hovering around body problems and the space between us, relationship tension has the potential to be healing Rainbow Medicine.

12 Symptoms Are Medicine from the Future

Quantum theory introduces a new idea, that of
imaginary time . . . not the kind of time we normally experience. But in a sense, it is just as real
as what we call real time. The three directions in
space, and the way the universe started out at
the Big Bang would be determined by the state
of the universe in imaginary time.
—*Stephen Hawking*[1]

In chapter 10, you discovered that working on your body gives
you insights into how to help groups. In chapter 11, troublesome
relationship fields appeared as Rainbow Medicine. These ideas
only scratch the surface of nonlocal medicine's potential.

In this chapter, I show how symptoms may be related not only
to communities in the present, but to future events and the past.
This statement is not as surprising as it sounds. After all, sometimes when dreaming, we feel as if we were in the past and the

future. Then, upon awakening, perhaps we realize that time is relative and too complex to understand with the everyday mind. Sometimes dreams in which we experience the future reorganize our paths and pull us forward, pressing us to do certain things now. Many of the people I have worked with dreamed of an older version of themselves with greater wisdom then the present self, and were thus informed by the "future."

Imagining Imaginary Time

Modern worldwide consensus reality is organized around clocks and forward-moving time. The phrase "yesterday at 5:00 P.M." makes sense to just about everyone; 4:00 P.M. today and 9:00 A.M. tomorrow are concepts with which people are familiar. However, some physicists use new concepts of time to explain the origins of the universe.

Cosmologists such as Stephen Hawking employ imaginary time from the equations of quantum mechanics—that is, from imaginary numbers[2]—to understand the nature of reality. On his website, Hawking explains: "One can picture it [imaginary time] in the following way. One can think of ordinary, real time as a horizontal line. On the left, one has the past, and on the right, the future. But there's another kind of time in the vertical direction. This is called imaginary time, because it is not the kind of time we normally experience. But in a sense, it is just as real as what we call real time."[3] (Figure 12-1 is mine.)

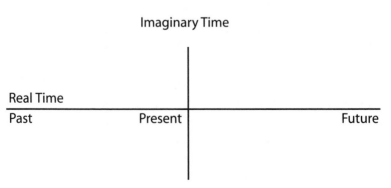

Figure 12-1. Real and Imaginary Time

Hawking, together with Jim Hartle, his colleague at the University of California in Santa Barbara, use imaginary time as a mathematical tool to bring together relativity and quantum theory. To envision a universe governed by both phenomena (relativity and quantum mechanics), it has to be born not from a singular point where time and space are both zero, but from a more complex version of time that allows continuous movement from imaginary spaces (those preceding CR dimensions) into "real" ones. (The concept of imaginary time allows scientists to avoid dividing anything by zero—which would quickly produce an impossible situation.)

In imaginary time, we are freer; we can turn around and even go backward. "This means that there can be no important difference between the forward and backward directions of imaginary time. On the other hand, when one looks at 'real' time, there's a very big difference between the forward and backward directions, as we all know. Where does this difference between the past and the future come from? Why do we remember the past but not the future?"[4] (See Hawking's public lectures, "In the Beginning of Time: 2002.")

Perhaps Hawking and Hartle were unconsciously following the directions of the great mathematician and physicist before them, Gottfried Leibniz, who (together with others) invented imaginary numbers during the European Renaissance in the 1600s. Leibniz defined the imaginary number "i" with the equation: $i \times i = -1$ and described i as the "Holy Ghost" of mathematics. Leibniz said that imaginary numbers are "a fine and wonderful refuge of the divine spirit—almost an amphibian between being and non-being."[5]

Though Hawking may not have been thinking of "amphibian[s] between being and not-being," using imaginary time to envision the origin of the universe restores time's nonconsensual aspect. For him, time has an imaginary component as well as a real one. If we can write time t as a complex number, that is as a number with both real and "imaginary" values, then we can say: $t = t_{real} + t_{imaginary}$ or more briefly, $t = t_r + t_i$.

t_i is the nonconsensual aspect of time, the "imaginary time." Its meaning is exact in math, but because it is imaginary, this meaning cannot be measured in terms of CR values. Thus, for example, $5i$ is not (measurably) greater or smaller than $3i$.

In any case, in the Hawking-Hartle theory, real time or t_r is zero at the beginning of the universe, but imaginary time, t_i, existed. If we think of the imaginary number as "an amphibian between being and not-being," we get a special insight into Hawking's view that "the way the universe started out at the Big Bang would be determined by the state of the universe in imaginary time." The new insight is that the universe began in nonconsensual reality, or Dreamtime, which is somewhere in between "being and not-being" in CR.

While controversy over the meaning of imaginary time rages in the scientific community, we can say with certainty that the mathematical concept of imaginary time is, in many ways, the metaphor for altered states of consciousness. Most shamans and therapists realize that events in life come from a time-like dimension of dreams. In other words, imaginary time is a metaphor for dreamland.

Every consensual concept is defined by complex numbers because everything has both real and dreamlike ingredients. For example, a tree is both a real fact in space and simultaneously a nonconsensual feeling for the observer. As another example, many casual references to time include both real and dreamlike aspects. To say that *morning* is your best time of day is to say that the real time from 8:00 until noon may be connected with the atmosphere of awakening or with the first light of day. *Evening* or *nighttime* is as real as it is poetic.

Thus imaginary time is a metaphor for *the atmosphere* we associate with the time measured by clocks. In imaginary time, we can move forward and backward in a nonlocal fashion as far as CR time is concerned, because imaginary time is not bound to a particular point in real time or space—only to a particular atmosphere. For example, we move into the future when we fear illness or death, but can go back to childhood and be a child, all in the space of a moment.

Nonlocality and Imaginary Numbers

In the world of math and physics, imaginary numbers have unleashed a lot of fantasies. Today, Heisenberg's interpretation of (the complex numbers of) wave functions in terms of tendencies is but one of at least eight possible interpretations of these imaginary numbers. My feeling about all the various interpretations of the math of quantum physics is that *all* possible interpretations are psychologically correct because each has something specific to say about the structure of dreaming. *Each interpretation of the quantum wave equation has a special, nonconsensual, and immeasurable psychological significance.*

For example, the standard interpretation—the one forwarded by Niels Bohr, Werner Heisenberg, and others (the so-called "Copenhagen interpretation")—sees reality as created, in part, by the observer's presence. In this interpretation, one cannot tell if the wave function is part of the observed system or of the observer.

In *Quantum Mind* I showed that Heisenberg's idea was a psychological truth: By marginalizing nonconsensual experiences, we create CR reality. For example, in dreamland, a given symptom may just as easily be represented by a monster or a gift. In CR reality, however, both are usually marginalized. We mostly speak of symptoms as mechanical or chemical problems (while perhaps suspecting, but rarely telling anyone, that we also think symptoms are both potential gifts as well as monsters).

In chapter 3, I discussed John G. Cramer's interpretation of quantum waves in connection with the idea of flirts. According to his interpretation, the quantum wave equation implies that observations are based upon the interaction of two quantum waves of equal strength and the same frequency, moving in opposite directions. He described the way these waves interact as similar to a "handshake" between telecommunications machines. Once this handshake has occurred, communication begins in CR reality.

I claim that we sense these flirts or "pre-signals," and then when consensual communication begins, we marginalize the flirts, just as we forget the buzzes and beeps that precede fax and e-mail connections once we are finally online. With flirts, we cannot tell whether an object wants us to look at it, or something in us wants to observe it. The point is, these flickerings happen in a subatomic world, a virtual reality, or an *imaginary time*. They are immeasurable nonlocal connections entangling our bodies and the world around us.

While Cramer worked for the U.S. National Aeronautics and Space Administration, he wrote a wonderful paper explaining his work.[6] He pointed out that the imaginary waves of physics (that is, the two conjugate waves of the quantum wave function) can be understood in terms of nonlocality. He said that because one wave moves forward while the second moves backward in time, nonlocality is implicit and basic to the equations of subatomic physics.[7]

Nonlocality refers to the nonconsensual aspects of objects and people that allow them to be everywhere, anytime, including both the past and the future. Behind CR reality exist interconnected nonlocal experiences that produce no measurable signals through the intervening regions. Thus everything, including a symptom, is created by immeasurable or imaginary experiences from the future and past—those tantalizing pre-signals that leave their tracks in our dreams, fantasies, and momentary lapses into altered states where flirts abound.

Backward Causality

To most people, *backward causality* seems less reasonable than forward causality. Most of us have felt that the past creates the present and future. Backward causality strikes us as contradictory. How can the future affect the present or the past?

Consider the following. If you think back in time from the present moment, you can imagine how past events seem to have been organized at least in part by what you are now doing in the present. Moreover, whatever you are involved in now is organized at least in part by the past. In the same way, the present moment and the things you are now doing are possibly influenced by the future of who/what you will become. Since these things in the future are happening in imaginary time, in dreamland, we can't measure or verify them in consensus reality (at least with our present methods). That is because CR verification would need to be capable of processing signals that reach out to the future so quickly that they go faster than the speed of light. That hasn't yet happened in our CR world, as far as anyone has verified.

Nevertheless, in dreams and in the mathematics of imaginary time, we certainly can and do speak of future-like events touching past-like events. In fact, our future deaths, imagined or experienced in a dream, reach backward to our feelings and thoughts today, creating fear, but also possibly detachment and freedom.

Let's explore backward causality to see how body symptoms may be organized by the future. The first step in this exploration is to reawaken your lucidity about tiny, nano-like experiences. Then we will focus on symptoms. In what happens next, I suggest that you use your awareness to pick up events—those evanescent flickers or flirts—that are very short lasting.

Exercise: Attention Training

To begin with, let's reawaken our awareness in a general way before applying it to symptoms. The first step in disciplining attention is to relax, take a couple of deep breaths, perhaps close your eyes or at least keep your eyes half closed. As you feel more and more relaxed, you'll notice a point when your eyelids are ready to open by themselves. Slowly opening your eyes, use your awareness to notice the first things that catch your attention. Catch and hold on to them. As you open your eyes, several things might flirt with your attention; let your unconscious mind choose which of these to focus on. What caught your attention? Was it a color, or an image, an object, a movement?

Let the thing that caught your attention explain itself. Let it "tell you" its meaning for you. Even if this interpretation seems uncanny to you, remember it. Make a note of this interpretation. For example, one reader, trying this exercise at night, saw the reflection of her lamp in the window. The lamp "said" to her, "I am here, there is light and knowing, even though you do not believe that things will be illuminated without your struggling to understand them."

Ask yourself if the interpretation you heard from whatever caught your attention might hold the answer to some larger question you have about your life. For example, as this woman pondered the "words" of her lamp, she remembered doubting her intelligence, thinking she had to learn more from books. The flirt-event suggested to her to believe in her own inner wisdom.

In what way could this message be from the future? Was the thing that caught your attention somehow an aspect of what you need or want to become in the future? Is this a flicker from a future self? Was the message perhaps an intuition coming from a wiser self who you might be one day? For example, the person who saw her lamp in the window felt it was an image of a "totally spontaneous person," one who just suddenly knew things without figuring them out. Such a person was what my reader said she was trying to become.

Now that your lucidity is awake, let us use it to work on body symptoms. The first step is to recall a body symptom that has troubled you in past years or which bothers you right now in the present. Choose one to work on. If you cannot choose one, let your unconscious mind choose one right now. This means trust your intuition about which symptom to work on. Alternatively, choose the one that first catches your attention just now, for whatever reason. For example, one of my readers chose pulsatile tinnitus, a ringing in her ears, to work on. This ringing increased when her heartbeat increased.

Relax and focus on your breathing. When you feel a bit more relaxed, gently turn your attention to your symptom area, feel it if you can (or if you can't, remember feeling it or see it), and let some aspect of the symptom catch your attention. Which aspect flirts with you in this moment?

What about your symptom catches your attention? Is it a feeling, movement, sensation, picture, thought, etc.? Let your unconscious mind choose which flirt to focus on, and hold that in your attention. Something in you will know. For example, my reader chose the "ping" sound inside her ear.

As you focus on this symptom, hold your attention on that special aspect that is catching your attention. What is this aspect like? Just let it work on you. Pretend this flirt can communicate with you. Feel it, imagine it, and when you are ready, let it "speak" to you. What is it saying? Listen and catch your flirt's very first imaginings. Let your flirt move you. Dance it. Hear it, visualize it. Then write down what it says. For example, my reader said that the ping reminded her of a the motions of a spontaneous young child who uninhibitedly bumped into whatever was around. "Ping, bang, oops . . . what fun!"

If you are having trouble understanding or accepting this message, ask yourself: What is the essence of this message? What is the root—its tendency, its basic significance? For example, my reader said that the essence of this message was to be free and childlike.

In what way is this message from your symptom a message from the future and an answer to your present situation in life? In what way do you already know this message but marginalize it? Why have you marginalized it? Does the message not coincide with the way you identify yourself today? Perhaps you are ignoring a deep part of your present and future self. For example, my reader said she had dreamed that as she grew older, she would be freer and more spontaneous than now. In the present, she felt inhibited and shy to move about in life the way she wanted to. She felt her dream was a "big dream" but that there were so many outer responsibilities in her present life that she had no time to be spontaneous.

Give the message or its essence a chance to transform you in this everyday reality. Let the future move you today. Instead of just leaving it in the world of dreams and body symptoms, move your hands, or if you can, get up and dance the message. Give yourself a few minutes to do this. Get its message, be the message, try to live it in this world, and realize how it was already there, trying to come forward, but was probably marginalized. Be the message-sender. For example, my reader said she got up and "danced in my room, floated, pretended I was a child, and thoroughly enjoyed myself." She let herself experience and imagine she was both very young and at the same time a free, older person.

How will your personal history and present behavior have to change in order to accept and integrate this body symptom, this message from the future? For example, my reader said that her family had brought her up very conservatively. To believe in her inner child would mean a radical life change.

In what way is your symptom message related to the whole world in which you live, perhaps to the whole universe? For example, my client said that the whole adult world around her was too anxious and serious. Her world needed more childlike fun and creativity.

Feel how living your message influences your symptom. Can you feel how your symptom is a kind of message coming from your future self? Perhaps the experience of your symptom was a message from the future, a nonconsensual tip from another time about how to live more fully now.

Symptoms Are "Receivers" Connected to the Universe

Nonlocal aspects of body symptoms connect you to the world. You can say that your body is a kind of radio receiver picking up messages from the future, personal messages coming from the whole universe. Symptoms give you the impression that the force of silence wants you to play certain roles in life.

Scarcely noticing these messages, your everyday self often moves along in life wondering why life seems unfathomable. We barely admit that we wonder what we should do next. Where do we go? What is the meaning of life? Why do I have a particular symptom? What should I do with my relationships? Even though we may be scarcely aware of these questions, the universe calls on us and answers them in terms of things that catch our attention, like body symptoms.

In a way, a body symptom is like a telephone call from the universe. The ringing asks, "Won't someone pick me up? I have something to say." Train your attention and pick up the phone. However, perhaps the problem is that you have no room for the phone on your desk. You need to make that phone part of your daily business. Make room in consensus reality for the ringing; otherwise, the business of daily life is incomplete.

Life and health are determined by what happens in imaginary time, in that realm that precedes CR reality, from which the products of dreaming emerge. Marginalizing imaginary time is not just a scientific problem but a public health issue. In relation to the practice of multidimensional medicine, consensus reality is worse than a virus—it is public enemy number one because it tells only a minute portion of the story of reality but claims it has the entire story. CR tells you that a symptom is worthy of consideration only when it bothers you, and then only in terms of sickness and health. Your body flirts and flickers are unimportant.

However, this serious health issue is one that can be resolved. Notice flirts from symptoms; they can be medicine from your future self. Catch and follow tiny body sensations before your ordinary mind judges them. That is the smallest and the biggest step you can take on behalf of yourself and your world.

13 Freedom from Genetics

... both genetics and morphic resonance are involved in heredity.

—*Rupert Sheldrake*[1]

If symptoms can be linked to the future, they are certainly connected to the past. Today, biologists call the known, statistically significant, causal connections to your personal history "genetics." Personal history is a combination of fact and fiction, genetics and myth. The story of where you come from, who your ancestors are, is linked to biological patterns you carry from the past.

If you want to know what your chances are of getting the diseases that troubled your recent and long-ago relatives, genetics is part of the answer. Its rules speak about your possible predisposition to certain symptoms.

In this chapter, I suggest how your genetics may be linked to your personal myth. In the next chapter I consider if, how, and why genetics can be controlled or reorganized—not only by poisons and radiation but also by the use of awareness.

137

We are programmed by our genes to be resistant to some diseases and get others. Yet awareness of guiding waves and myths may change all this programming in unexpected ways. These new ideas lead to a psychogenetic method that is based on the interaction between genes and dreams.

Cell Biology

So far in this book, we have been thinking of our bodies on the physical level mainly in terms of elementary particles and atoms. Now let's think in terms of *cells,* those basic units of living systems which we might call the atoms of life.

Cells are small. Ten thousand human cells are needed to cover the head of a pin. Each of us has about 75 trillion cells. Each cell contains a set of chromosomes with the heritable genetic material that directs our development. This material comprises the "genome," the instructor of your physical development.

These chromosomes contain the genetic code, which is composed of DNA—billions of atoms linked in the form of two coils, entwined as a double helix. Stretched out, the DNA located in just one tiny cell of your body would make a thread about two meters long. Unwinding that chromosome, it appears at first like a string, all looped up around itself.

Our genetic material, our genome, is similar to the genomes of other life forms, from fleas to gorillas, bacteria to bears. A chimpanzee's genome contains between 95 and 98 percent of our genes. We know that when the cell is not in the midst of division or replication, our DNA is dispersed throughout it. However, during cell division, DNA coils and folds itself into threadlike chromosomes that split and carry the genetic code to next generations and into the future. The number of chromosomes per cell is constant for each species. Humans have 46, that is, 23 pairs of chromosomes, and each pair is shaped like a double helix.

Scientists believe that our human DNA has existed for three and a half billion years on this planet. Genome accidents originating from inside or outside the body injure the DNA and hence influence

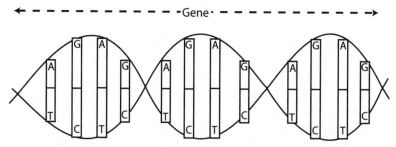

Figure 13-1. Genes Are Locations on Intertwined DNA. A, G, T, and C, the nucleotide bases, form a "word" that spells out genetic information.

the reproduction of cells in the future. According to present theories, natural selection uses these accidents or mutations to sift out mutants according to their fitness. Only the advantageous errors survive. In this picture, nature operates like an automobile company. It produces many cars, tries out many motors. The best motors are best as far as power and efficiency are concerned; the worst are accidents leading to less positive or even dangerous results.

In the late 1800s, Gregor Mendel discovered the basic rules governing genetics. He explained, for example, how it is possible for grandchildren to look like their grandparents instead of their parents.

Today, we know that Mendel's "unit of inheritance," the gene, occupies an area on the chromosome. In 1953, Watson and Crick discovered the physical and chemical structure of the DNA, the double helix. They realized that DNA (or deoxyribonucleic acid) is the backbone of the chromosome. DNA, a long, thin continuous molecule, is a chain of minute subunits known as nucleotide bases. Genes were found to be specific sequences of these base pairs. Four different kinds of bases exist in the chain—adenine, guanine, cytosine, and thymine. Their sequence in a gene determines its properties.

DNA appeared to be a sort of spiral staircase, and the genes were the steps in that staircase (see figure 13-1). Twirled chromosomes of DNA, with gene locations on the helix, are sketched in the illustration. The gene is composed of thousands of base pairs.

Human Genetics—and Our 100,000 Genes

The 23 pairs of chromosomes in our genome determine a lot about our lives. For example, if the 21st pair has three instead of two chromosomes, then Down syndrome occurs.

Genes from our parents' ancestors determine many of our physical characteristics. Characteristics such as height have a relatively large genetic component. Others, such as body weight, have a relatively large environmental component. Still other characteristics, such as blood type and the antigens involved in the rejection of transplanted organs, appear to be entirely genetic, meaning that no one environmental condition is known to change these characteristics.[2]

Our human genome contains approximately 100,000 genes, of which about 4,000 may be associated with specific diseases. Susceptibility to various other diseases also seems to have a genetic component. These diseases include diabetes mellitus, Alzheimer's disease, multiple sclerosis (MS), schizophrenia, Huntington's disease, malaria, several forms of cancer, migraine headaches, alcoholism, obesity, high blood pressure, and bipolar disorder.

To decipher the genetic code, scientists must unzip the strands and explore how they are templated.

Though some physical characteristics are largely determined by genetics, we are not entirely programmed. The way in which you deal with your physical body, where you live, and what you eat influence your life span. Further, the manner in which you feel and think also has feedback connections to your genetics at the biochemical level.[3]

Nothing about you is entirely determined by one factor or one set of factors. A human trait that is primarily hereditary, such as skin color, can be changed by how you live and by environmental influences (e.g., sun exposure). On the other hand, any trait sensitive to environmental influences, such as weight, has genetic factors involved. The fertilized egg cells from which you grew contain programs for your basic constitution, yet there are many possible outcomes depending upon how you live your life.

Heredity is not destiny. Genetics gives us an overall view of

Mendel's Genetics

Genetics research inspires both wonder and terror, depending upon whether it is used to cure diseases or clone new and "better" species. At present, genetics provides a map of the human world, but not the details. We see the continents but not the streets. As research progresses, the field hopes to uncover the individual street maps as well.

Gregor Mendel, an Austrian monk in the 1860s, became the parent of modern genetics by claiming that a factor called the gene was the basic unit of inheritance. He did not yet know what genetic material was or where it was located, but from his study of peas he realized that it determined the inheritance of a particular characteristic or group of characteristics. His theory promised to resolve the underlying mystery of heredity and evolution.

He discovered that genes obey simple statistical laws. To explain these, first remember that an offspring comes from two animals or plants of the same or different races/breeds, varieties, species, etc.

Mendel's law states that cells of all offspring can be divided into two categories. Half of the reproductive offspring cells transmit one parental unit and the other half transmit the other parental unit. This separation of alternative characters in the reproductive cells is now known as Mendel's first law. It is also called the principle of segregation and can be used to predict what happens in nature when single pairs of alternative characters are observed through several generations.

Take the following case, for example. A single gene (R) determines a flower's color. R is the dominant gene which causes a flower to be dark in color, and r is the recessive gene for a light-colored flower. Since R is "dominant" when paired with r, the flower is still dark in an Rr combination. Only in rare cases is rr found, a double-recessive gene pair, which produces a light flower.

Thus, two parents with Rr genes can produce offspring according to a basic law of probability easily expressed in a "Punnett square."

	R	r
R	RR	Rr
r	Rr	rr

RR offspring, a 1:4 probability, are double-dominant dark. There is a 2:4 probability of having an Rr offspring (also dark), and a 1:4 chance of an rr offspring, which will be light.

what might occur, but it does not tell us about the individual "accidents" in our cells or who will bump into us to change our lives. Life is a mixture of chance *and* determinism, making it unpredictable.

The results of a questionnaire, handed out by a friend of mine at a recent genetics conference, showed that most of the scientists who responded think that what happens to us is 50 percent genetics, 50 percent environment. "Environment" is a collective term for the psychological impact of your upbringing, the people you grew up with, the food you ate/eat, the schools you attended, and so on.

Nonlocal Influences on Genetics

An agreed upon, unifying paradigm connecting genetics, medicine, and psychology with environmental effects does not yet exist.[4] We know from previous chapters that our dreamland sense of the atmosphere around a person or organization is nonlocal. The force of silence, the quantum fields we sense in dreamland as "the environment" touch everything in a nonconsensual (i.e., largely immeasurable) way. In the same vein, genetic accidents (i.e., sudden changes in the atomic and molecular structure of our genes) and the resulting natural selection of the fittest are also connected with nonconsensual fields.

In a previous chapter we met biologist Rupert Sheldrake and his proposed morphogenetic fields. His idea is that natural selection depends upon what has been learned in the past. According to Sheldrake, the fact that an earlier generation learned new things makes it easier for us to learn them today. (We see evidence pointing to this principle each time the Olympics are held and new records are set and new feats, previously undoable, are accomplished.)

I suggest that Rainbow Medicine is a unifying paradigm connecting psychology, medicine, and the environment. As quantum medicine, it studies the effect of quantum nonlocality, the patterning of our pilot waves, and the songlines of our dreaming on our genetics. We know that our genetic code can be changed measurably by real physical factors such as radiation, which damages chromosomes. Further, during replication, unexplained mistakes in reproduction ("accidents" and mutation) can damage genes. Such accidents during the process of replication are partly responsible for illness and aging.[5]

What appears as the disturbance of an atomic or molecular structure in CR reality may be due not only to known physical causes, such as toxins, radiation, or even fluctuations in gravity, but also to the immeasurable basis of such causes—what I call the force of silence. We know that almost all symptoms, explained by medicine in terms of specific consensual causes, are experienced in dreams in terms of mythic imagery. I call this phenomenon the dreambody. What is experienced as an accidental illness can appear in dreams as a pattern trying to manifest in the person's life. For example, one of my clients, sickened by radiation resulting from an atomic reactor leak, dreamed a friend of hers had changed the whole world for a particular reason.[6]

Feelings and relationships play both a disturbing and a healing role in our overall health and sense of well-being, a finding that has received much support in the CR experiments of several interrelated disciplines exploring psychosomatic processes. Therefore it is reasonable to imagine that nonconsensual fields, pilot waves, not only interact with our personal myths but also affect our genetics and the whole of our biophysical chemistry.

Your Genetics

Before learning how dreaming interacts with your genetics, let's begin with some personal fundamentals. Consider your own genetics. The following general questions about your genetics may help you get in touch with the experience of your personal history, of people and fields influencing your present life. Don't worry about complete or "correct" answers. These questions are meant to simply start you thinking about your inheritance.

- Consider aspects of your body you feel you may have inherited from your parents and grandparents. (If you don't know one or both of your biological parents, imagine them. In my experience, the imagination of these people has often turned out to be very close to reality.) Let your answers be a mixture of fact and fantasy. Where did you get your weight, body build, skin tone, hair color, and eye shape? Is your posture linked to a family member?

• Do you fear getting the diseases of those who preceded you? Where do you think your heart and vascular system came from? Who had cancer, diabetes, colon trouble, arthritis, osteoporosis?

• Do you use any medications? If so, are they linked to your family history? To which side and person in your family?

• With whom do you associate some of your talents? Where did your most fascinating attributes come from?

• In what way are you a living piece of history? In other words, imagine how your problems carry not only the genetics but also parts of the unsolved problems of your parents (or imagined parents) and ancestors. How might you fit into your family or cultural history? How are you something new, and at the same time, a story of the past trying to complete itself?

In some way, you are a crucible in which history is trying to transform itself, and your body problems may be at once an anchor to the past and a solution for the future.

Exercise: Dream Gene Playhouse

If you consider only how your CR genetics are linked with your history, you can begin to imagine a kind of historical theater that looks to me like a picture used by the Mayo Clinic (see figure 13-2). This diagram, however, only traces our localized genetics. It does not address the infinite creative possibilities linked with this map. We will address those possibilities here. To begin with, allow yourself to experiment, to *dream into* and to rearrange family figures or imagined family figures.

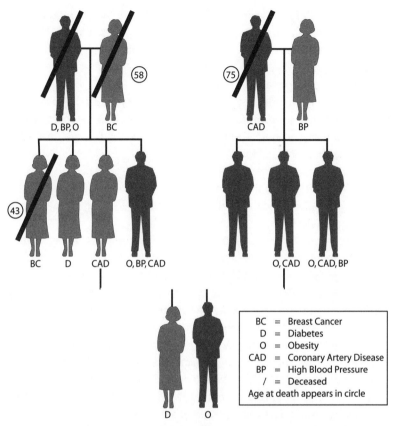

Figure 13-2. Inheritance Map. This inheritence map traces how diseases such as cancer, diabetes, obesity, and heart and vascular problems are passed down in history.

Pretend you are at the theater. Imagine that you are sitting in your seat in the audience, making yourself comfortable. Look up at the stage. As the curtain opens, the players in your playhouse come forward, and they are the family you came from.

Imagine your sibling(s), parents, and grandparents on stage. (Again, if you don't know your family, imagine them.)

Place these figures on the stage in any way you feel they should be placed. For example, you might have to place yourself in the middle.

You can use other living family members—use whoever feels important to you. As the play goes on, you can add to your psychodrama people who have already died or are about to be born.

To do this in the most helpful manner, take a few minutes right now and tear up a sheet of paper into many pieces. Write "Mom," "Dad," "Grandpa," etc., on separate pieces and place them on a "stage" in front of you. Take note of your First Act—that is, the way the pieces of paper are placed.

Now that you have put your pieces wherever you feel they belong, let your creative mind, the force of silence take over. Play. Let the pieces of paper move around. Add new figures if you feel they are needed until the theater feels done.

Take a pause then and reflect about what happened on stage. Your final act is probably a combination of your physical and psychological inheritance as well as psychological changes trying to take place within you.

For example, one woman said she was surprised at her final arrangement. In act one she felt she was a "throwback" to her dad's dad, whom she resembled. She felt closest to him in many ways and furthest from her sister. She also said that she had apparently inherited the physical diseases of her father's father. In her final act, my reader added a female social activist whom she admired, realizing that this heroic feminine figure was somehow present. Though her parents had courageous qualities, she felt more connected to that feminine heroine. To her great surprise, she placed herself and this heroine alone in the middle and finally had the other figures join and watch the center of the stage. This explained to her the separateness she felt from her family of origin but also made her want to tell them all about her development.

Creating your dream gene playhouse is a form of play; it happens spontaneously, in response to reading these pages, and may have been based upon flirts, intuitions, and the force of silence. In CR, you are a part of your theater, and in dreaming, you are the entirety of all that is on stage. You are the sum of all parallel worlds, including your past, and you are co-creator of the future. In fact, what you might call "your" creativity—the spontaneous rearranging of these figures—is a manifestation of what the force of silence is trying to create.

Does changing your genetic theater in fantasy change your symptoms and genetics? In the next chapter, I suggest that this change may occur by showing how your playhouse is linked with your genetics as well as your personal myth.

14 Genetic Backaction—How Dreams Influence Genes

If you look deeply into the palm of your hand, you will see your parents and all generations of your ancestors. All of them are alive in this moment. Each is present in your body. You are the continuation of each of these people.

—*Thich Nhat Hanh*[1]

To sum up, although each form of thought of the essence is an appearance, it also reflects a reality that is, however, always dependent for its existence as well as for its qualities and properties on broader contexts and deeper levels.

—*David Bohm*[2]

Real CR fields such as electromagnetism, gravity, temperature, and air pressure influence the body in measurable ways.

However, immeasurable, personal nonconsensual fields, feelings, dreams, and fantasies always accompany those very real forces. The subtlest field is the force of silence. You feel but cannot easily verbalize its intent until it has unfolded in dreaming or appeared approximately as an event in reality.

In chapter 13, we considered genetics and its possible relationship to our somatic and psychological experiences. In many ways, we are products of our parents, ancestors, and ghosts of the dead. In this chapter, we experiment with "backaction": how awareness affects intentional fields, genetics, and symptoms. What you feel touches not only your momentary body states but also your inherited gene expressions, your present life, and the life you inadvertently pass along to others. In other words, your feelings influence the future, just as all the generations that preceded you are touching you now. What we call mutations and genetic accidents are a possible connecting point between genes and dreams.

How Psychology May Influence Genetics

To consider how psychology might influence our genetics either directly or through apparently accidental mutations, consider the similarities in the structure of fantasies and gene expressions.

Psychological patterns that appear to be inherited, or at least passed down, can be found in childhood dreams. These patterns are narrations or recountings, a counting or numerical idea, as are points on a line. In any case, stories and dreams are lines or strings of basic images, portraying shared human phenomenology, which Jung called archetypes or archaic images; they are found in the myths and fairy tales of people from all over the world.

According to Jung, the archetypes are inherited characteristics, "seeds," behind images or clusters of images. These recountings (the German word was *erzählung*, which originates from "number") are a psychological parallel or counterpart to genetic expression, which also is a patterned account occurring on a string (chromosomes) of countable inherited units of genes.

Based upon the many hundreds or thousands of childhood dreams or recountings I have heard from both children and adults (claiming to remember their childhood dreams), it seems to me that such dream recountings are assemblages of units predicting our physical and psychological behavior. This predictability makes them roughly analogous to the predictions about our bodies which can be made knowing our biological genetics.[3]

Almost a century ago, Jung pointed out that standard collective images, such as those of the great mother, the divine child, the ruler, etc., are found in cultures the world over. He called these images archetypes and implied they were the analogies of biological patterns such as instincts. When a series of these images appears in folk stories, it is called a saga or fairy tale. When such a series appears in a person, it is called a dream.

When many people believe in a given tale, it becomes a saga. Over time, sagas lose their personal and local identification and evolve into collective myths. Jung believed that the mythic images seen in dreams are inherited phenomenological blueprints coming from the experiences of our ancestors.[4] Jung's work evolved from his own studies and from the ideas of Freud, who was more biologically oriented and who thought mainly in terms of intrapersonal drives such as the sex drive or the death wish.

When I was a psychology student at the Jung Institute in Zurich in the 1960s, one of my teachers gave me a copy of one of Jung's most interesting (yet, as far as I know, unpublished) works, an unedited manuscript called "Kinderträume" ("Childhood Dreams").[5] Based on the dreams reported in that manuscript, Jung points out that repetitive childhood dreams predict the future occupation of the individual dreamers.

My research generalized this finding. I discovered that those childhood dreams not only predict the future occupation of dreamers but their future body experiences. For example, a woman's childhood dream about a lion scratching at the curtain of a window not only symbolizes the lion-like power she met as a child and will meet and develop later in life, but also symbolizes the itchy or scratching feeling that did appear in a lifelong chronic skin problem. The lion scratched the window curtain in the same way the adult scratched what turned out to be a chronic skin irritation.

That lion is an "inherited" instinctual pattern, a psychological pattern also associated with the dreamer's childhood home. In any case, symbols (such as the lion or curtain) in childhood dreams may be thought of as units along a string, a count, or an account. The essence, or Jung might say the archetype, behind clusters of such units (such as a lion scratching a curtain) might be thought of as "psychological genes." Both genes and archetypes appear in dreams and behavior as clusters of symbols and patterns of behavior.

Childhood dreams, such as the lion dream, are dreamland expression of personal myths—long-term patterns derived from "psychogenetic" codes. Further, like genes, sections of these patterns are sensitive to the everyday mind, or transformable depending upon the imaginations of the dreamer.

Assuming this connection between our genes and dreams, we may suspect that early childhood dreams are expressions of underlying patterns or archetypes, which I shall call "dreamgenes." In biological reality, our genetic expression appears as units of inheritance; in psychological reality our long-time patterns appear as symbols in childhood dreams.

The Influence of Consciousness on Dreams and Genes

Changing people's relationships to their psychological inheritance, to their dreamgenes, is one of psychology's main tasks. Whether as a Jungian, Freudian, Gestalt, Adlerian, or process-oriented dream worker, therapists interact with dream figures and childhood memories of patients by using, following, analyzing, and battling them to create *coherence* between the everyday mind and the totality of the human soul. Bettering your relationship to those early figures changes your experience of life.

From a process-oriented perspective, here is where the parallels between psychology and medical biology end: at the point of transforming genes, both biological and psychological. Whereas biology and medicine speak in terms of advantageous or disadvantageous consensus-reality events such as healthy or ill genetic combinations, process-oriented psychologies speak in terms of consensus-reality events and dreamland processes including the potential meaning and purpose of problems and events.

In other words, from the CR viewpoint, a particular arrangement of genes and dreams may be judged as good or bad. But in dreamland, illness or accidents can be seen as highly meaningful events, often pointing to life-enriching experiences.

An example is a person who suffered radiation poisoning. Her problem was diagnosed as serious and predicted to be fatal within months. However, she dreamed she had been "freed from the most dreadful prison." Her dream told her that she was not sick, but being freed. After working on that dream, she decided to free herself from particular life circumstances. Twenty-five years after she was supposed to have died, she told me that she still had many body problems, but felt as free as could be. Was this luck?

Anecdotal evidence gives me the impression that the physical future of dreamers actively interacting with the dreamland aspect of body experiences is no longer predictable. Getting in touch with the deepest part of yourself, your pilot wave, makes the path feel certain in dreaming (e.g., freedom). You feel better, more whole, and sometimes even detached from the symptom process in consensus reality.

The job of psychology and Rainbow Medicine is to follow the deepest path of an individual: to explore, relate to, co-create, recreate, reconstruct, or adapt to the configurations of their dreams and subatomic body states. Biological medicine working at the CR level alone aims at changing troubled or disturbing genetic combinations as if they were aberrations instead of meaningful occurrences.

Nevertheless the following question remains to be answered: If certain medical procedures can repair some genetic problems, can psychology do the same? If so, how might relating to the dreamland context of real events interact with body experience and those rejected genetic expressions? To answer this question, let's explore these possibilities in terms of your experiences. To introduce this exploration, I discuss different approaches to working with dreams and body situations, and then I apply these approaches to working with your psychogenetic situation.

Childhood Dreams—Dreamgenes in Conflict

As an example, let me speak about my own childhood dream and see how it connects with my physical genetics. The first dream I can remember occurred when I was four years old. In the dream, I was a little boy polishing my father's car. As I polished away, a big growling bear came by. "Grrrrrrrrr!" it said. He scared me so much, I ran into my father's car for protection. Relentlessly, that bear got in the car too and continued to chase me; I was running for my life in ever greater circles around that car until I woke up.

The basic units or dreamgenes seen in that dream are my father's car and the bear chasing me. Both the bear and my father's car are linked to feelings I had about my family. My dad was a hardworking, good-hearted, predictable, quiet guy. His philosophy was "Don't do much in life, just enjoy the moment, work, pay your bills, and settle down. Polish the car."

But the bear is very different. I associate the bear energy with my mother's energetic, unpredictable nature. As a child, I wanted to be more like my father, but my mother's energy has always chased me. She never seemed to know what to do with her energy. (And I never know what to do with mine!) In my dream, the bear seemed to disagree with me; the bear was angry I was polishing the car—that is, angry that I was identifying only with my father. Even as a child I knew the bear was upset with me for having marginalized his seemingly wild energy.

In a way, polishing the car is part of the father gene in me, and the bear chasing me is part of the mother gene in me. Though my parents basically got along with each other, their energies conflicted inside *me*, and this childhood dream shows how my dreamgenes are in conflict with each other.

Childhood dreams typically show a combination of genes from both parents, and often a conflict of some sort. By favoring one of these genes (the car), we marginalize the other (the bear). Marginalization comes about spontaneously and unconsciously. By identifying ourselves with only some of our parts, we create an identity based on marginalizing other parts. These marginalized parts almost always turn up as symptoms or as scary dream figures seeking attention.

By identifying with my father, who marginalized his own wildness, I was chased about by bear-like energies and pressures. One of my earlier chronic body symptoms that later improved was wild swings in blood pressure. (The men on my father's side of the family typically suffered from blood pressure problems.)

Here is another example of dreamgenes at work. I am reminded of a client who suffered from lung problems. He could not remember a childhood dream but recalled a first memory of his mother, who was being mean to him. He said his major body symptom was emphysema, probably due to smoking. He worried about this symptom because his father had died of lung cancer.

He associated his mother with the mean feeling of cramping in his lungs. She was always bitter and cramped. To work on his memory, he shape-shifted into the figure of his mother and explored her essence. To his surprise, behind her meanness was coldness, a sort of detachment and a "quietness" about relationships. This warmhearted, "motherly" man realized he had spent his life trying to compensate for his mother's coldness, and that now, from the world of her essence, he found a sort of cool detachment and freedom from always being nice to people, and he was much happier.

Best of all, his new behavior affected his lungs. Being cooler and less attached to others relaxed his lungs immediately and resolved the cramping. After his work with this dreaming process, he got better, and his medical doctor later thought the diagnosis of emphysema had been incorrect.

Exercise: Dreams, Symptoms, Genetics

Childhood dreams seem to show psychological as well as biological/genetic components. The next exercise gives you a chance to explore these ideas for yourself, to see how your dreams, genetics, and symptoms are connected. You will need to recall either the first childhood dream you can remember or, if you can't remember one, the very first event you can remember. Then you will be asked to explore methods of recreating the dream (or dreamgenes) in a theatrical fashion and relate it to your body experiences.

Write down the earliest dream you can remember (or the first childhood or teenage memory). If you can recall several dreams (or memories), choose the most powerful of these.

Sketch two simple figures from your dream. If you dreamed (or can remember) only one figure—such as a bird flying or falling—consider the second figure as the one implied in what you are doing. For example, if you are flying, consider the sky or the ground as second images.

Could these two figures be related to your mother and her family or your father and his (or your imagination of these people, if you never met them)? For example, the car in my dream is related to my father and his father (who gave him that car), and the bear is connected with my mother's energy.

Sketch or draw an outline of your body. Now sense your body and ask yourself with what parts of your body these dream characteristics are associated. First just meditate and sense your body, and then sketch these figures on your body sketch. Do you have symptoms located where you placed your dream figures? For example, I have my dad in my elbows, where I also have dry skin, and I have always had a sense of pressure in my chest.

Once your figure is complete, work on your childhood dream. Ask yourself: Which is the most difficult dream figure for me today? For example, that bear's animal energy is still the most difficult part of myself to manage.

After identifying this energy or figure, act out this figure, remembering your playful, childlike nature. Use at least one of your hands. Enjoy yourself. Be a child and act out that figure.

While moving and making sounds, feel deeply into the figure and try to get to the essence of that figure and its energy. This exercise has no one correct response. We are looking for a feeling. We are searching for the basic tendency of that energy, before it became an image and became so dramatic. For example, my bear's energy was essentially the tendency to move freely in a oneness with nature.

When you are ready, shape-shift into that figure and live in the time and the space of that essence. Get into this parallel world and just be there. Live there. Try to live in the world of that essence. For example, I imagine living in the world where things just happen in the oneness of nature and there is no second-guessing, no evaluation, no weighing and measuring.

Try to experience this world as fully as you can. Do you see images and hear sounds?

From the world of the essence that you are now in, look back at your childhood dream or memory and explore how you would recreate all or part of that dream. For example, I would make my father more like the essence of the bear, more fluid in his ways, less mechanical.

As this essence, interact with, change, influence, or recreate that dream. Dream the dream on or create a new resolution or story, using the same or different figures. In other words, look back at the dream or memory and think how you would influence it as this essence. Take time and actually tell yourself a story. Make it up. Let the essence world create things.

Act this new story out and then write it down. Create a theater. Use music or movement, rhythms or songs, poetry or art. Use your imagination, have an open creative mind, something like a child. For example, in my recreation, the bear that was chasing me becomes a dancing teacher who dances with me and my father.

Give yourself plenty of time. This is an unpredictable and creative act on your part. Then look at the new story that you created and ask yourself: Why did I not create or dream this story in the first place? What was your original dream working on when you were a child? Was it reacting to your tendency to marginalize one part and favor another?

What circumstances did not allow your essence to unfold as it has today? How have you, or could you, change? What basic elements of you are changing? What basic dreamgenes? What attitudes in your conscious mind?

Let's connect these dreams and fantasies with your body. Take a moment and reexperience your resolution and the feeling that came out of that story that you just created. Feel it and express it with your whole body in movement. Dance it with your hands and your arms and your whole body, if you can. Notice how your movements influence your chronic symptom area. Notice what kind of effect occurs in that symptom area.

How might this story influence what you are feeling and doing these days? For example, just now I am editing this manuscript, and I can imagine doing it in a more dance-like manner.

Reflecting on the Results

In your everyday life you probably see your body symptoms as problems that you want to change. Marginalizing a parallel dream-world element (such as the bear) in everyday life corresponds to experiencing (or projecting) that bear as an irritating friend in relationships and/or as body symptoms. Not marginalizing that particular parallel world makes you more coherent. Psychologically, your attachment to your everyday CR identity provokes your pilot wave, which is a sum of parallel worlds, to accentuate that parallel dream world element. If you irritate one of your parallel worlds (the bear) in order to maintain your identity, that particular parallel world stands out in your awareness in the form of a symptom.

For example, the more I marginalized my bear's parallel world, the wilder my blood pressure fluctuations became. With increased awareness and coherence, you are less likely to view your genetics as either good or bad, but as signposts showing you the way to your whole self. This dreamland viewpoint is different from Darwin's CR principle of survival of the fittest. In dreamland, all energies and essences are held in equal value.

The point of this exercise is to discover various perspectives and to see the value in each. You interacted with your dreamgenes, your psychogenetic map, and perhaps you got to its essence, the force trying to co-create your universe. In a way, the marginalization and irritations of your childhood dream also are linked to your cultural history and your family, and the energies (values, characteristics, attributes) they have accepted or marginalized.

Your symptoms express how the force of your dreaming reacts to the boundary conditions you needed in order to maintain your particular identity. Coherence changes these conditions. From the dreamland viewpoint, CR genetic expression linked with illness offers potential opportunities and gifts.

Backaction and the Path with Heart

From the essence viewpoint, from the force of silence, your personal myth is partially represented in dreamland as clusters of dream figures, and in biology as genes. All these figures are superimposed, like the various colors of the rainbow, creating a diversity of possibilities in life. They all sum up to an overall glow, your personal myth whose essence is the force of silence. Your timeless self, like the pilot wave, is nonlocal. Marginalizing one of its overtones stresses that tone (that dream figure) and makes that parallel world a troublesome and *symptomatic* one for you in everyday reality—as a source of body symptoms.

In effect, by accepting your various tones, you create a sense of harmony and a new theater we might call the *path with heart*. If David Bohm and Richard Feynman were alive today, I can imagine their comments. Feynman is saying, "Yes, the path with heart: that is the sum of all possible histories, all those virtual realities, all the possible paths you have taken in parallel worlds." And I hear Bohm saying, "Of course, and once you use your awareness on your ship, you create a backaction with your pilot wave. That's what I meant when I said that a particle can influence its quantum wave functions. It directs you, and you direct it."

Using Bohm's image of backaction in which a ship interacts with radio waves informing the ship where to go, we can understand better how awareness might affect the body. Without awareness, your body problems are local CR symptoms with possible genetic causes. Awareness, sensitivity to the dreamland and essence levels of symptoms, changes everything. Awareness allows you to discover and surf your pilot wave, so that your whole body feels better. Through feeling more in touch with your whole self, your life reorganizes. Not only do your dreamland parts interact differently, but all your body parts interact in new ways.

Either directly, or indirectly through other body parts, dreamland and essence surfing experiences unpredictably influence the genetic problem localized in the space and time of your cells. That's how dreams influence genes. The original somatic genetic disturbance is either relieved or becomes less significant as new multidimensional life experiences emerge.

III
AGING: CHEMISTRY, BUDDHISM, AND ENTROPY

15 Aging and Buddhism

All are clear, I alone am clouded.

—*Lao Tse*[1]

At age 24, I began my therapy practice in Zurich. One of my first clients discovered quickly how little I knew. He was the first person I had worked with who was over the age of 60. He complained of feeling severely depressed and asked if I knew how to cure depression. I told him I did not. Under these circumstances, I suggested he see someone else or tell me exactly just what he was experiencing.

"I'm depressed!" he yelled, furious with my ignorance about the subject. I gently persisted, "What's it like?" Luckily for me, he took my suggestion and began by responding with a long moan, "ohhh," and putting his head in his hands as if it were a load of bricks. After groaning for a few minutes, he looked up, and seeing his hands in front of his tearful eyes, he suddenly froze. Staring at the palm of one of his hands, he gasped the words, "Oh, no! *M!* That's *memento mori!*"

Surprised at his statement and not knowing at all what he was referring to, I mumbled, "What does that term mean?"

"Remember death!" he exclaimed. Before I could say anything, he went on. "Yes, death, death, death!" Then, as if hit by something terrible, he wept bitterly. A few minutes later, he explained that the "M" on the palm of the hand signified remember death in his Swiss-Italian part of the world. Death is always present, he somberly instructed me. To my amazement, after some minutes of crying and remembering, he announced his depression was gone. He said he felt suddenly closer to the priests he had detested in his childhood and that "something spiritual happened." He left.

It took me years to understand that. Later, reading the teachings of don Juan Matus, I began to understand. Don Juan said, "Death is your best ally." Death tells you, when nothing else makes sense, that only the touch of death is crucial. Nothing else is as important. Detach from the rest.

Remembering death, remembering aging, means that time passes. Get closer to what is meaningful. The CR body gets older and eventually dies. It sounds like an obvious insight, but most people try to forget it, as if time did not exist, and insist on identifying with earlier appearances. By holding on to past identities, by saying, "Oh, no, I am not aging," you marginalize your shape-shifting nature. A one-sided view of life is toxic to the spirit. One-sidedness can be depressing and irritating to your body. Scary as it is to relinquish the view that we are here forever, remembering death can lead to a freedom from the constraints of time and space and everything else in this CR world.

We have been looking at symptoms from various perspectives in this book. In part 1, I focused on working with individual symptoms, and in part 2, on their relationship to the world and ancestral dreamgene patterns. Now, in part 3, I want to explore how awareness affects the aging process. In this section on aging and death, individual symptoms will no longer be our focus but the *clusters* of symptoms associated with the aging process. In essence, we will examine the somatic effects of how we view the passing of time.

Physical Aspects of Aging

Following (see table), I list some of the physiological changes associated with aging and hint at some of the dreamland experiences accompanying those symptoms. The psychological experiences are merely suggestive; they come from experiences I have had with people working on their aging process. Let me say that the psychological material in the table is meant to be merely suggestive. Moreover, the physiological components are not facts that fit everyone, but only averages. Not everyone is affected the same way by aging.

For example, aging affects the brain; over the years, most people lose some of their memory capacity. The ability to learn new things is reduced, though exactly how much is debatable. The typical older person with memory loss forgets others and eventually herself.

When I first studied psychology, I heard about a psychiatric category called senile depression, referring to older people who become quieter and sit around more than before. However, most of the research at that time was done with people who lived in institutions and nursing homes, and it did not include folks living more independent lives, people who were mentally and physically active. Today, it seems clear to me that older people can be depressed not because it is a characteristic of the aging process, not because of biological changes, but because of psychological problems such as broken relationships or (like the client mentioned earlier) because they have not culled the meaning of aging and death.

Many heart problems produce noticeable symptoms. When the heart weakens, many people dream about doing less or being more detached in what they do. However, a few dream that they need to start on something completely new. This reminds me of the aging shaman, don Juan, who, racing over the mountains, his young apprentice (Carlos Castaneda) trailing, claimed his power was due to his detachment or his "not-doing."

Aspects of Aging

Organ or System	Natural Effects of Aging
Skin	Loses thickness and elasticity (wrinkles appear). Bruises more easily as blood vessels near surface weaken.
Brain and Nervous System	Loses some capacity for memorization and learning as cells die. System becomes slower to respond to stimuli (reflexes are duller).
Senses	Become less sharp with loss of nerve cells and poor circulation.
Lungs	Become less efficient as elasticity decreases.
Heart	Pumps less efficiently, making exercise more difficult.
Circulation	Worsens, and blood pressure rises as arteries harden.
Joints, Bones	Lose mobility (knee, hip) and deteriorate from constant wear and pressure (disappearance of cartilage between vertebrae results in old age "shrinking").
Muscles	Lose bulk and strength.
Liver	Filters toxins from blood less efficiently.

Accelerating Factors	Dreaming Processes
Process accelerated by smoking, excessive exposure to sun.	Sense of self and boundaries change or weaken.
Process accelerated by overuse of alcohol and other drugs, repeated blows to the head.	Forget the moment, detach from self and even human history.
Process accelerated by smoking, repeated exposure to loud noise.	Stop looking at and listening to self and others, connect with infinity.
Process accelerated by smoking, poor air quality, insufficient exercise.	Stop breathing, hold your breath, and stop time.
Process accelerated by overuse of alcohol and tobacco, poor eating habits.	Becoming less powerful, more sensitive to change.
Process accelerated by injury, obesity.	Less ability to follow social intent, sense of "Thy will be done."
Process accelerated by injury, obesity.	Discover skeleton, that part of person which is old or infinite. Experience self as disappearing.
Process accelerated by insufficient exercise, starvation.	(If food is no problem) Let go; give in, let things happen.
Process accelerated by alcohol and drug abuse, viral infection.	Don't take life for granted; connect to events with awareness instead of throwing life away.

Circulation problems can be due to blocked arteries. Gradual clogging is difficult to detect until the blockages create symptoms in organs not getting enough blood. Yet people who sense a circulation problem (such as clots) often say that they experienced a kind of "Stop" sensation in their bodies. Many hear the message, "Stop doing what you have been doing."

The aging liver filters fewer toxins out of the blood over time. People with liver problems of all kinds often speak about changing their lifestyles and personal history. They tell stories about how they have played with life unnecessarily, considering it a given, instead of a temporary gift. Many used addictive tendencies and drug-induced altered states of consciousness to gain access to spiritual experiences. Liver problems redirect our awareness to gain access to hyperspaces without the use of toxic substances.

While traditional medicine focuses mainly on preserving the physical form, Rainbow Medicine sees death as just one of the many worlds parallel to everyday life. From the quantum view, from the force of silence, we are a combination of death and life. In everyday life, we may marginalize death to such an extent that it spooks us and we keep it in the background of everything we do. However, from a dreamland perspective, death is only the end of our identification with certain characteristics and the beginning of a new potential to open to new vistas.

Defining Aging

Terms such as *life, love, nature,* and *aging* point to multidimensional experiences. The CR component to aging usually refers to the deterioration of our physical body. Our appearance changes; we become shorter, more hunched, gray, balder, wrinkled; hearing, seeing, and sensing are dulled; and memory is less acute. Aging usually means progressive physiological decline. Psychologically, the part of us that imagined it could live forever is constantly shocked at the deterioration. At the same time, aging can mean freedom from one's self and one's social concerns.

The Biophysics of Aging

Recent scientific research into aging is aimed at inhibiting the aging process in cells. As already mentioned, each cell carries the body's full genetic code in the DNA stored in its nucleus. DNA controls the cell's activities and responses. Every time a cell divides, the DNA replicates. To prevent and correct mutations, enzymes within the cell nucleus constantly monitor the DNA. Nevertheless, some cell-level mutations in the body's somatic cells (tissues like skin or muscles, or in organs, glands, etc.) go undetected, and when the cell divides, this cellular damage is replicated in future generations of that cell's divisions. The cell's DNA repair system itself undergoes aging and is less able to do its job. In time, then, the DNA with errors is passed on to new cells, creating more and more errors. Those microscopic errors in that one cell finally add up to tumors or body deterioration and aging.

In addition to the fact that the repair system itself goes downhill, another major cause of DNA damage is free radicals. These are reactive, electrically unbalanced molecules produced during normal metabolic processes involving oxygen. To neutralize these electrically unbalanced chemicals, the cell uses various compounds known as antioxidants, among them the vitamins C and E and other chemicals found in fruits and vegetables. Antioxidants preserve foods (and gas, oils, etc.) by inhibiting them from turning rancid. Nevertheless, free radical damage does occur and is thought to be one of the mechanisms of aging. It has been found that humans have much higher levels of antioxidants than shorter-lived species.

A nonconsensual definition of aging is that it is awareness of the growth of the death of who you were. *Aging is the death of the marginalizer,* the one who was able to ignore the dreaming, little flirts, and sensations. Eventually, the whole of life becomes one of those strange flirts or sensations that can no longer be avoided.

Unbelievable as it may seem to some of us, no one knows exactly why the CR process of aging occurs. Most biologists argue that aging is a part of the evolutionary pattern. According to this thinking, evolution is organized by natural selection; those people whose genes give them long life pass on those genes. The human race has never cultivated genes endowing health and strength into old age because (in CR) nature seems (and people, too?) to have focused on using genes for growth, development, and reproduction. Therefore, in old age, scientists tell us, our genes are predetermined to let us down.

In consensus reality, the passage of time causes aging. It seems as if we have a genetically predetermined life span. Few of us will live beyond the age of 119, if that. Life's finite nature is supposed to be due to a combination of genetic and environmental characteristics. As with all symptoms, Rainbow Medicine approaches the aging process as an awareness process and as a CR medical situation that can be partially prevented and treated.

Aging and the Force of Silence

In chapter 6, I spoke of life in terms of physiology, as "life is that which breathes and moves." The metabolic definition of life was connected to having a CR identity linked to a permeable boundary. The genetic definition added biochemistry and the environment, making life an evolutionary process with adaptations in response to the world around us. In biophysics, life is order, and entropy wins over order, finally destroying life.

Rainbow Medicine's definition of life also includes the force of silence, or nature's subtle intent that connects existence to quantum mechanics and parallel worlds. In Rainbow Medicine, CR aging is body deterioration; in dreamland, aging is a subjective, individual experience; and in the essence world, aging is but one facet of the force of silence.

For example, many people complain about aging in terms of fatigue and sagging body parts. The stomach, shoulders, breasts, testicles, and other organs begin to sag. Without exercise, the body relaxes. Instead of working against sagging—which can be done with exercise, for example—the experience of sagging can be revelatory.

I remember asking a middle-aged woman in one of my classes about her experiences of aging. She told me she felt that sagging was the outstanding experience of aging in the moment. She followed my suggestion about not just talking about aging but experiencing her description of it and, while standing, slumped forward. I suggested she use her awareness and follow whatever wanted to happen. She slumped further, then stopped for a moment to comment that if she let go, she would give in to the force of gravity. Then, sinking to the floor, she made a discovery.

The Earth was there for her, holding her up. The Earth, she explained, "was like God." Sagging turned into a spiritual experience for her, as she let herself sink into the hands of God. When she could no longer carry herself, when she let go, she sensed something else was there for her. Sagging is a mechanical problem linked to aging, yet in dreamland aging turned into something divine.

My suggestion is to use your awareness. Understand that words like *aging* and *depression* are terms that have CR meaning but negate dreamland experiences, which can be transformative. You, dear reader, should ask yourself how you define aging. How do you experience aging right now? Instead of staying with that description of aging (as if it explained something), take a moment and *feel into* that experience.

As an experiment, let yourself sink down into dreamland and be overtaken by your aging experience. Shape-shift and let aging happen. Let your body experience and explore your present experience of aging.

When that experience has unfolded its full expression, imagine an image of a person with your unfolded body feeling. For example, if you are tired and find yourself relaxing, imagine a relaxed person. Let yourself be that person to discover the force of silence trying to manifest in you right now. Enjoy that experience and discover its meaning.

Aging is a collective name for an experience, still essentially unknown, that is trying to enlighten you about your nature! From the viewpoint of nonconsensus reality, dreaming, not aging, exists. This viewpoint is close to that of major spiritual traditions such as Buddhism.

Basic Buddhist Ideas on Aging

Aging is central to some spiritual traditions such as Buddhism. The brief summary of Buddhism which follows leaves much to be desired, but I must include it because some of Buddhism's main ideas are closely related to both the scientific and spiritual dimensions of Rainbow Medicine.[2]

According to legend, Buddha spent his first 29 years in a protected and privileged living space. In his 30th year, he left that protected existence and entered the everyday world. The first thing Buddha saw was "The Four Signs." The first was the "Old Person," the second was the "Ill Person," the third was the "Dead Person," and the fourth was the "Holy Person."

His first step toward enlightenment after leaving the palace was seeing the Old Person. Then came illness, death, and the Holy Person. This story represents many things, but within the context of this book, the protected space in which he lived the first part of his life might be understood symbolically as naïve youthfulness. At 30, he awakened to the existence of aging, social issues, and pain.

Then Buddha followed the path of the fourth sign, the Holy Person. Meditating under the Bodhi tree, he freed himself from consensus reality with the realization that all things are interdependent and empty. Buddha realized that life is suffering due to attachment for material things and pleasant states of mind. Buddha discovered that suffering and craving could be resolved through right action, right living, and right concentration (using the Eightfold Path[3]).

Meditating and following the rising and falling of inner experience led the Buddha to outline several general principles to relieve suffering. The first Buddhist principle is impermanence—*amitya.* Nothing endures. Notice that all experiences arise and fall away; they come and go. *Everything is process.* The wave forms basic to quantum physics also imply that the universe is essentially a wave in process. All is in motion.

The second Buddhist principle says that everything in CR is empty—*sunyata.* The word *empty* can be understood in many ways. I like the interpretation of the Zen master from Kyoto, Fukushima Roshi, who speaks of emptiness in terms of openness and creativity. Emptiness suggests that, at the essence level, events are full of creative spark but devoid of any permanent form or content. For example, a chair is empty in the sense that *chair* is a consensual idea that marginalizes the essence of that chair which, as a CR object, transforms over time. In this sense, consensus reality contains emptiness.

Another example: You probably think of yourself as a person in everyday reality. But naming anything negates its underlying motion, its ongoing fluidity, and pins it down to being one thing. However, even CR science now knows that there are no firm things or objects that are stable and permanent. In this sense, all is empty. Taoists use another way of describing this emptiness. They call it the Tao which cannot be said.

In Buddhism, things become what we know them to be in CR through their interdependence. For example, we know a symptom is a symptom only because of the interdependence of everyday reality with history, science, pain, and suffering. Any one symptom is interdependent upon all things. Without any one of those elements, a *symptom* would be something else.

For example, in a culture that had no concept of symptoms as we think of them (a signal of something gone wrong), they would not exist. What we call cancer exists only because we assign a certain configuration of attributes to an accelerated growth process. Assign another set of attributes, and you've got an entirely different experience. The underlying emptiness of CR reflects the principle that *all meaning is assigned; nothing is intrinsic.*

The third Buddhist principle, *Atman,* means "no-self." We as

171

individuals have no permanent ego or identity, if for no other reason than the CR self grows and dies.

Aging As a Parallel World

The Rainbow Medicine view of aging includes a mixture of scientific and spiritual ideas, of measurable and immeasurable realities. We are all aging, and at the same time, aging is an empty term for an unknown and mysterious process. In dreamland, aging can be represented by many parallel worlds. In dreamland, regardless of your CR age, "you" are both a baby and an old person, living and dead, yourself as well as many other figures. You are a constellation of many universes.

In CR, you seem to be a single person only because these other universes are marginalized. Only the sum over *all* your potential histories, your death, your life, your childhood, your old age—and everyone else's—is the total you. The sum of the stories of all your parts makes sense. One world by itself is insufficient and leaves you feeling nervous, as if something were missing in life.

My wave summation diagram pictures a summation of these various worlds, a sum that amounts to your timeless path with heart.

Exercise: Working with Aging Symptoms

In addition to working with the overall experience of aging, it can be very helpful for some people to work with specific aging symptoms. A useful way to do this is to identify a specific body symptom that you feel might be connected to aging. Take a moment and do that now. If you have several symptoms, let your unconscious mind choose which body symptom or experience (possibly due to aging) to work on in the moment.

Feel that symptom, or notice its effect. In what manner does it reduce your earlier state of physical health? For example, is your sight weaker? Does your body sag so that you are less strong? Is

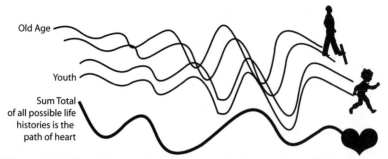

Old Age

Youth

Sum Total
of all possible life
histories is the
path of heart

Figure 15-1. Wave Summation. The sum of aging and youthful worlds and other parallel experiences or rhythms of the pilot wave.

your skin changing? Is your heart or stomach or sexuality less vital in some way?

Instead of resisting, analyzing, or only medicating this aging symptom, notice *it.* Don't just think about it in a rational manner. Rather *feel into* the symptom (or imagine the feeling you would have if that symptom increased). Now let that feeling experience increase a bit more. Allow the process of that symptom of aging to unfold itself. Simply notice how, in your imagination, you might change as time goes on. The point is not just to lament these changes, but to notice and allow the changes to occur along the lines of your experience and fantasy. For example, if your eyes are weaker, imagine what it is like to see less, to be less able to focus on the world around you.

Use your inner awareness and track what happens as you go even more deeply into this aging process. Hold your attention on the deterioration happening in your imagination, and, while experiencing it, find the basic tendency, the ever-so-subtle intention behind this development. Let your first flickering thoughts about this arise and catch them. For example, the essence of your weakening eyesight might be to no longer look outside, but instead to notice inner tendencies and follow them. The essence of weakening eyesight might be taking the world less seriously, and—like Jacques Lusseyran who was blind—learning to sense life differently.

Explore the world of this essence. Every time you think about aging, notice it, remember death, and remember that, in a way, both *aging* and *death* are empty—they are no more than the names assigned to unknown experiences. Leaving whatever stability you may have had in your life until now, explore letting old age occur.

Let impermanence lead you through emptiness to a path with heart beyond time and space. Is this essence experience, the path with heart, somehow the sum of your old age and some essential part of your youth?

Remember the suggestion of the shaman don Juan about what he called "the path with heart." It is the path a very wise and old person takes; it is a path free of ambition and other people's ideas. This path makes you happy. Other paths eventually make you curse your life. If you are not on the path with heart, there is no affront to you, or anyone else, in dropping what you are doing to find it. Aging is part of the path with heart when you see it as empty and explore its mystery.

16 Why Free Radicals Kill

Now we know how the electrons and light behave. But what can I call it? If I say they behave like particles I give the wrong impression; also if I say they behave like waves. They behave in their own inimitable way, which technically could be called a quantum mechanical way. They behave in a way that is like nothing that you have ever seen before. Your experience with things that you have seen before is incomplete. The behavior of things on a very tiny scale is simply different. . . . The difficulty really is psychological and exists in the perpetual torment that results from your saying to yourself, "But how can it be like that?" which is a reflection of [an] uncontrolled but utterly vain desire to see it in terms of something familiar.

—*Richard Feynman*[1]

How you treat aging, genetic problems, cells, and symptoms depends, in part, on what you believe treatments do. For example, if you think of aging in chemical terms, you might think of rusting metal and deteriorating bodies. Then you would have to take antioxidants because these prevent "rust" (as I discuss below).

But if you view aging not only from the viewpoint of chemistry and biology, but also include psychology, suddenly rusting and the wearing down of parts is linked with more than oxidation. From this new rainbow viewpoint, aging, rusting, and oxidation are not just CR facts, but mental imaginings, metaphors associated with unresolved cravings. If this sounds to you like Buddhism's suggestion that suffering comes from attachment, then you are correct. In my view, here, in the midst of electrodynamic chemistry, is another magical point where physics, psychology, and spiritual teachings converge.

Today's biological viewpoint sees us as a moving collection of about one quadrillion cells. This is definitely the world of "the ten thousand things," to use Taoism's term for consensus reality. Looking at ourselves with a microscope, we appear to be a bunch of cells, and about half the genetic material in each is also found in a banana. The fact that the basic components of life—the things that make us human—are only about 3 percent different from a chimpanzee might make you uneasy, or perhaps convince you that, in general, you are "the other." You and I are interdependent with bananas, apes, and everything else.

The Senescence Factor

From previous chapters, we know that cells regenerate and repair themselves because the DNA code constantly separates and duplicates itself, recreating life. The cell divides in the process of mitosis. Were it not for accidents, this replication process would go on forever and we would be immortal.

In 1961, Leonard Hayflick, an American microbiologist at the University of Pennsylvania, performed an experiment on human cells. He found that body cells replicated 50 times before they no longer divide and begin to senesce (age). To this day, no one can explain why they stop replicating after 50 times. Cell biologists call the unknown factor limiting the reproduction of cells "SF"— short for senescence factor.

There are several SF theories. The first is the autoimmune theory, which proposes that autoimmune reactions occur when our defenses, normally meant to attack foreign things from the outside that endanger the body, attack the body itself. In psychological terms, we defend our individuality against attack, but in so doing, we go too far and begin to attack ourselves as well. Autoimmune reactions are a bit like self-hatred in psychology.

Free radicals are a second SF theory. Toxins and accidents damage the DNA, and free radicals are one of the internal toxins that create genetic accidents and aging. Simply stated, free radicals are substances with an unbalanced electric charge; they have a free, or extra, unpaired electron. These unbalanced radicals attack the DNA, drawing electrical charge from the DNA, thereby disturbing cell chemistry. The result is that the DNA no longer replicates as well. Thus free radicals create mutations and are part of the senescence factor. Free radicals are considered contributors to many diseases, including diabetes, arthritis, Alzheimer's, and heart trouble.

Free Radicals and Buddhism

Buddhism and biochemistry agree on one point: Attachments create suffering. If you remember that the free radical electrically craves a positive charge, then what the chemist thinks of as a free radical is a metaphor or symbol for that part of us that craves what it is missing. One way to understand the chemistry of free radicals is to think of cravings, attachments, longings, and hungry ghosts. For example, remember how you behave when you are very hungry. Better yet, remember times when you eat, not because you are hungry but because of some unknown craving. Without awareness, your craving makes you forget the agony of the living beings such as animals, fish, and birds, that you must eat. Survival of the fittest! Longing, when unattended to and unsatisfied, cancels awareness and makes us potentially dangerous to ourselves and others.

Free Radical Oxidation

In the sketch below, the free radical molecule on the left has a couple of unpaired electrons and a resulting negative charge. Imagine being this radical, searching for a charge to balance yourself. You would be hungry for some positive charge to make you feel better. You might even break the law to ease that craving. Free radicals are like thieves.

In chemistry, these free radicals create a process called oxidation, in which one or more electrons is removed from a substance. The free radical molecule that no longer remains negatively charged oxidizes by combining with genetic material (on the right) that will no longer work properly after it picks up extra electrons.

The free radical oxidizes when it loses its electrons. You know about the process of oxidation because of what it does to food. Oxidation turns oil and butter rancid and changes iron into rust. Antioxidants like vitamins C, E, and A work against oxidation by neutralizing the free radicals. When the free radical sees these vitamins or antioxidants around, the radical goes off with them instead of the DNA.

Hungry free radical, with two unpaired electrons.

The positively charged molecule is endangered by the free radical which is about to come closer and combine.

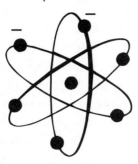

Free Radical

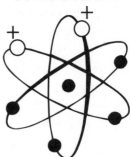

Positively Charged Molecule

Figure 16-1. Free Radical Oxidation

Just as free radicals are part of the senescence factor, so are cravings. Cravings and addictions wear us down and ruin the body. The more one-sided you are, the more your heart races, the more your stomach produces acid, the more you burn and long for *something*, the greater the stress factor, and the less well you feel.

Spiritual attitudes and detachment approach this problem and are a kind of psychological antioxidant against craving, just as vitamin C is a physiological antioxidant. Buddhism, Taoism, and other related traditions are "antioxidants" in the sense that the practice of their tenets is directed toward neutralizing cravings to enhance detachment and overall balance. It is almost fashionable today for medical people to recommend meditation as an antidote to stress.

Exercise: Into and Beyond Cravings

If we view our chemistry theories (as we do in physics) as metaphors and dreamland patterns, then free radicals are stressful attitudes, one-sided cravings. For example, a workaholic attitude might make you crave relaxation—or, more likely, crave a drug that will help you relax. One-sided strivings seek their own resolution.[2] Unfulfilled one-sided lifestyles crave balance. (Worldly attachment is often balanced by suicidal under-eating; subtle depression may be balanced by overeating.) As long as cravings are unattended, fulfillment happens unconsciously, can be self-destructive, and is never satisfying.

A Rainbow Medicine view of addictions is that they are a kind of psychological radical chemistry. Though addictions point to unknown parallel worlds, they also increase the addict's separation from consensus reality. In a way, the addict becomes addicted to being split—to experiencing a sober world separated from drugged experiences. Either one or the other is affirmed but not both together.

In Rainbow Medicine, the resolutions to symptoms such as addiction are embedded in the symptoms themselves. In the next exercise, solutions to cravings are found in their parallel dreamland experiences. Finding the essence of the addiction can ameliorate some addictive tendencies. For example, the essence of a sex addiction might be a loving attitude. The essence of alcohol could be letting go of everything. You may find you are attracted to a particular cookie because of its sweet taste or its creamy texture. You may smoke because exhaling gives you the chance to let go of something.

In finding the essence of addictions, you will be studying the psychology of craving. Imbedded in the experience of any craving is the dynamic of projecting power onto substances such as sweetness or letting go, while believing that you have no such power available *within* yourself. Focusing on this idea that you are projecting something about yourself onto an object or substance will lead to the essence of that particular addiction.

>*When you are relaxed and focused enough to work on yourself, name one of your addictive tendencies.* It may be challenging for you to think about addictive tendencies, but think of and name a tendency you might have toward abusing some substance or food. After you have the name, ask yourself, "What is the deepest unfulfilled wish behind this tendency?" For example, your need to be loved might be linked to an addiction to sweets. Many who feel un-mothered and who are persistently self-critical are addicted to sweets.
>
>*When you are ready, explore your craving.* Ask yourself: What physical feeling does this one-sided craving produce, and how does it affect my body in its most extreme form? Which organs does the addictive tendency involve? Which muscles might it affect? What body parts does my neediness disturb? For example, does it bother your lungs or head, stomach or muscles, skin or eyes, throat or mouth, etc.?
>
>*Feel your craving, and imagine someone who might represent the object or substance you are craving.* Who is this person? What kind of person is she or he? What is her or his world like? Let your creative mind send you an image of a person or even a mythic being that personifies the thing you crave. For example, you might see some spiritual or social figure, some eccentric or hypnotic figure, some sweet or very mean person.
>
>*Now let's go further into the nature of the image.* What is the essence of this symbol or imaginary being? What is its core, its deep-

est essence? To find the essence of the craving, it might be helpful to imagine what this image was before it became so amazing or so dramatic. Become the personification of the craving and feel its world. Then get to who it is in its deepest core, before it became one-sided or extreme in its behavior. That is the essence of the craving. Make a new image out of that essence. Keep searching for the essence until you feel relieved. For example, if the craved object is a cookie and its personification is a sweet motherly figure, the essence of that motherly figure might simply be a loving presence. An image of this presence might be a nun, for example.

Explore the world of that essence, that satisfying quality. Stay in that world. Then look back at your ordinary self and try to value both the essence world and your CR self.

The essence of your cravings, lived in everyday life, is a kind of antioxidant in the sense of balancing a craving. Notice how it changes your sense of your body to live the essence rather than indulge in the craving for it.

Between You and Your Craving

Addictions are linked to your one-sided identity. You have somehow decided that you do not have the same power as whatever you crave. Of course, you do have the power of that thing, but instead of accepting that power, you unwittingly give it away to the substance. In a way that may be hard to accept, you and the substance (or object or act) you are addicted to are one, or better yet, you share the same essence. The essence is a field that unfolds into your one-sided nature and that of the substance—but is neither. This essence is beyond polarization, beyond attachment; it simply is. It is not bound to any thing or person.

Cravings accentuate the aging process. They are robbers of your multidimensional powers. That is why even if the addictive substance is momentarily satisfying, in some way it is slightly depressing because of its implicit belittling effect. You look down on yourself and up to the addiction, giving away the power of a hyperspatial, dreamlike, or magical field between you.

What you thought of as a craving is, from a more sentient viewpoint, a field of power, filled with what physicists might call virtual particles.

Cravings are like electric fields, full of virtual power, something you can feel deep in yourself or notice drawing you towards others. The essence or power behind a craving or an addiction is another description of the force of silence that connects you to all things. Marginalizing this power splits that field into parts; it splits you in two, leaving you craving that which you believe you don't have.

Integrating your cravings gives you a greater sense of wellness. Marginalizing your power creates more "electricity" between you and the thing you are after. In principle, such a polarization influences your virtual fields, your quantum chemistry, the number of free radicals in your blood, and even the aging process.

Whether virtual particle theory and the extra free radicals due to addictions are understood as metaphors for your psychology or as medical facts, you need not wait for proof of consciousness's backaction whereby awareness influences quantum wave functions and electrochemistry. For today you can feel the immediate benefit of getting to the essence of your cravings and discovering some of your greatest powers.

The Buzz That Counts

Now that we have at least an intuitive sense of Richard Feynman's quantum electrodynamics, I want to ask you a question: How do you think he ever arrived at a such an imaginative theory?

If you are a physicist, you might answer that the overarching laws of physics governing the interactions between charged particles allowed him to replace electric fields with virtual particles. After all, they do not disobey any laws, and there is nothing which seems to forbid them.

However, if you are a therapist you might answer differently. I for example think he imagined virtual particles between charged

Magical Powers in Quantum Electrodynamics

Finding the essence of an addiction makes you feel better and may influence your free radical biochemistry. Biochemistry and quantum electrodynamics may explain why.

Richard Feynman, the father of quantum electrodynamics (QED), saw the space or field between objects attracted to one another as filled with the power of magical particles. He said that electric fields—such as those found between electrons and protons (and between any electrically unbalanced objects, such as free radicals and DNA)—can be seen not only as electric fields but also as what he called virtual particles.[3] The electric field that surrounds an atom's electrons and protons explains why atoms stick together. An atom or molecule with a negative charge (because it picked up an extra electron) seeks combination with another molecule with a positive charge.

Instead of speaking in terms of electric fields between molecules and atoms, Feynman developed the concept of virtual or imaginary exchange particles.[4] Feynman explained that two charged particles, like two electrons, repel one another not because of an electric field between them but because this so-called field actually consists of zillions of virtual particles or photons bumping into one another. He saw these virtual particles, or photons, as being absorbed by and emitted from each electron. Because the virtual particles bump into one another, the electrons repel one another.

In other words, two charged particles, such as two electrons, repel each other not because of their electric field but instead because that field consists of their virtual particles bumping into one another and the electrons.[5] Better yet, these virtual particles are

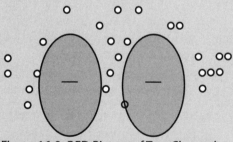

Figure 16-2. QED Picture of Two Charged Particles. Charged particles create, eject, and absorb virtual photons (shown as small circles), which then bump into the larger particles, keeping them apart.

conceived to be created out of nothing; they come out of the electrons and get reabsorbed by them before they can be seen, measured, or weighed.

According to QED, the tiny exchange particles or virtual particles go forward and backward in time. We can't tell which electron first popped out a virtual particle to bump the other electron. We only know that in the quantum world, there are uncertainties about time and space and measurement. These uncertainties make it impossible to measure virtual particles, because they exist for too short a time.[6] This view of large charged particles, like electrons, surrounded by a bunch of exchange or "virtual particles" replaces the idea of the electric field. Likewise, in biochemistry, the concept of electric fields surrounding atoms and electrons can be replaced with that of virtual particles.

objects because at one time or another, all of us have a subtle sense that the things which attract and repel us strike us as important. Slang expressions in English hint at the flirt-like bumps and bangs given to us by other people and objects. For example, if someone attracts us, we might say she is "smashing." There is even a song entitled, "I Get a Kick Out of You." Consider the expressions, "You are a knockout" or "That great movie was a 'hit.'"

The basic idea is that there is something like virtual particles flying between you and the things you feel attracted to and repelled by. Those particles are a dreamland buzz, usually discounted by the everyday mind. Getting in touch with the power of that buzz can not only free you from addictions, but can transform everyday life into magic. Each time you feel drawn to or repelled by something, every time you merely intend to do something, notice the essence-buzz of little "hits," the common ground of activity connecting you to that something. The buzz you feel may be a universal shared dynamic, holding our world together, giving you the sense that as you reach out for something, it reaches out for you as well. In other words, your intent is nonlocal, and it is not yours alone.

17 Telomeres Spell the End

Everything changes, nothing remains without change.

—*Buddha*

Biochemistry and psychology are clear about the detrimental effects of imbalance. One-sidedness makes you crave the other side until you become a "free radical" in every sense of the word. Eventually you develop addictive tendencies toward the very powers you feel you cannot have, and you project those powers onto other people and substances. Addictions threaten your health and accelerate the aging process, thereby threatening to extinguish your identity.

We humans are driven, biologically and psychologically, to affirm, expand, and eventually detach from our personal history. When our sense of personal history and identity begins to diminish or transform into a detachment from the past, fear of death often arises.

One way or another, everyone gets older. In relation to the senescence factor, biochemists discovered—and, in my opinion, also projected—a quality of detachment from personal history they named telomere destruction. In this chapter I show how this aging factor troubling our DNA is mirrored in the legendary Zen story of the ox herder. Once again, Buddhism helps explain the biochemistry of aging.

Consensus Reality Methods of Fighting Aging

In chapter 16, I mentioned how the experimental biologist Leonard Hayflick discovered that human cells divide 50 times before dying. Why 50 times? It seems as if we are genetically programmed to die. Not only stress, addictions, and cravings, but radiation, food toxins, and this genome program contribute to our demise. We know we can retard aging by avoiding radiation, food toxins, and the stress that comes from attachments to people, substances, outcomes, and possessions. We can eat less to detoxify our bodies; we can exercise, work on our cravings, explore new attitudes toward symptoms, and create healthy lifestyles. According to CR research, taking vacations and reducing daily stress levels reduce the mortality rate due to all diseases.

Telomeres and Personal History

Recent research suggests that "junk" DNA left around in our genome after replication contributes to aging. Junk DNA is pieces of our genetic programs no longer needed. When I first heard about this "junk," I was reminded of a perennial psychological/ spiritual message: let go of junk, drop old baggage you no longer need.

Biochemists tell us that, over time, aging destroys telomeres, the caps on chromosomes, which we have demonstrated might contain our personal, cultural, and human species history. The destruction of these telomere caps exposes the ends of DNA to degenerate after replication, and the degenerated DNA then contributes to the junk in our genome.

The Ends of Our Genetic Substance

The free ends on linear DNA molecules are unstable. As they recombine during the process of mitosis or cell division, they deteriorate more rapidly than the rest of the chain. To get around these and other problems, our bodies (specifically, the eukaryotic cells) have learned to cap chromosomes at both ends with specialized structures called telomeres.

The DNA polymerase enzyme responsible for replicating the genome during cell proliferation has difficulty copying the ends of the DNA molecules, so the end molecular sequences tend to deteriorate in the new copies. To retard this process of shortening the genetic material, nature put on caps. Nevertheless, because of the difficulty maintaining these caps, after many cell divisions, cell death ensues. In short, destruction of telomeres contributes to aging.

Physical exercise, healthy food, vitamin supplements, and detoxifying the body through eating less help deter this process. In addition, a body enzyme called telomerase, when specially added to the cells that have aged the most, tends to rejuvenate them. Telomerase is thought to be an anti-aging material; the chromosomes of young people are longer than older people and have more intact telomeres supported by more telomerase.[1]

Telomerase, like all catalysts, is something of a chemical village elder. A catalyst enzyme brings together two or more parties, called reactants in chemistry. The enzyme does this very quickly by creating an environment in which reactions can take place hundreds of times faster than normal. Yet the catalyst is not changed by the reactions it catalyzes. The catalyst is like an ideal mediator. Though independent, its presence speeds up the process in a beneficial way.

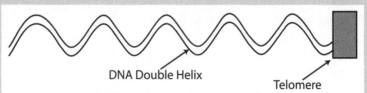

DNA Double Helix

Telomere

Figure 17-1. Genetic "Cap." Essentially linear DNA is capped at the end with a telomere.

Our chromosomes have a linear architecture that tends to fray at the ends. Animals and plants also maintain their genomes as collections of linear molecules, the ends of which also fray easily. Not all life forms have linear genomes, however; bacteria generally maintain their genome as circular molecules.

After working with people for many years, I imagine the psychological parallels of this shortening of DNA—this shortening of the code for our personal histories. On the one hand, we all need our personal histories and identities, and it's a pleasure to protect those identities as much as possible. But identifying with one fixed image of ourselves limits our potential.

The shortening of the telomere is a fact, but like all scientific formulations, it is also a symbolic statement about our psychology. In this case, we are dealing with the psychology of letting go of personal history. In dropping personal history, you let go of who you have been. Over the age of 25, psychology is coherent with the biochemistry of aging. Your genes carry the software or code dictating who you are (or were), and that code gets less significant as you age.

In earlier chapters we saw how genetic formulations can be reflected in childhood dreams, personal myths, and the experiences of body symptoms. In chapter 15, we saw how chronic symptoms can be linked to parents and ancestors. Now let's explore how shorting personal history allows you to let go of the dominating presence of your personal myth and also may result in reducing your identification with body symptoms linked to your ancestors and to aging.

Your Personal History—Who Are You?

Who are you? Your answer to this question is a large part of your personal history. How do you define yourself? Are you descended from native peoples, Africans, Latinos, Koreans, Japanese, Chinese, Europeans? What is your race? Your color? What is your belief system? Do you ascribe to a religion or spiritual tradition? If you have a particular one, try naming that, at least to yourself.

Identify yourself in other ways (or refuse to identify yourself—that position also is an identity). What is your sexual orientation? Economic class? Health situation? Are you a woman, a man, a bisexual, transsexual, homosexual? A working-class person? Upper-middle class? How old are you?

Your personal history is entwined with very specific characteristics. The first person or two you choose as a partner in an adult relationship seems to be part of your personal history (in the sense that she or he often resembles one of your parents or family-system caretakers). In everyday life, you may have had conflicts related to your personal history when you chose someone of the "wrong" gender, "wrong" race, "wrong" age to be your friend or partner. When you take actions that conflict with your personal history, everyone and everything around you rebels.

In growing more aware of yourself and others, you are likely to become more aware of your personal history in all its aspects: the love and comfort of it (or not), as well as the conflicts and disappointments it holds. Perhaps you will consciously seek to abbreviate it by detaching from it. You may become aware of how defending your identity against attack actually supports an old personal history, or creates a new one. Only death, the fear of death, or the fear of forgetting and losing memory bluntly call into account the whole process of creating and maintaining personal history.

Dropping personal history is part of the teachings of don Juan.[2] He speaks of the life and death of his parents. He tells his apprentice that his parents were agonized by what had happened to them and to their people in history. However, according to don Juan, the saddest thing was that they could not see themselves as *generally* human, free of the drive for revenge that accompanied their strong identification with one particular group. Don Juan says life is too short to have any one identity, and death is our only true advisor.

Ox-Herder Pictures—How to Remove Personal History

The Zen ox-herder pictures found on temples throughout China, Korea, and Japan give many insights into the gathering and removing of personal history. These sketches are folk pictures, fairy tales showing aspects of detachment from personal history within the context of Zen practice. These pictures represent typical phases of life and, for me, have wider significance than their application to Zen practice.

Though usually seen as stages in taming the restless mind, the ox-herder pictures also symbolize the process of working with all psychosomatic experiences—and eventually dropping personal history. I am grateful for permission to use the sketches found on www.buddhanet.net[3] in explaining the following.

1. What is missing in my life? How can I solve my problems?

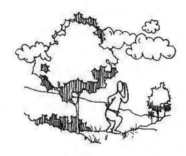

In the first picture portraying this legend, you see someone beginning down his path, searching for the way. Imagine it is you. Perhaps you are pondering questions such as "Who am I? How did I get here? What is life all about?"

In this picture you are lost in nature, lost in your own nature, your own vegetative environment. Perhaps you are looking for what a meditation practitioner might think of as the lost dream, the lost body, the missing dreambody. At this point, you are in a state of confusion, seeking the path to the future.

2. Oh, there are signals in the Earth.

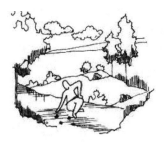

In the second picture, you find footsteps, perhaps even a path, indicating that something/someone has gone before you. In the earth, there are basic signals from the past. Perhaps you have discovered subtle body signals or other kinds of tracks within yourself.

If you follow these signals, you come across powers that may have run away without you. A Zen practitioner might identify these powers in terms of her "restless mind."

3. Ah-ha! There is my power!

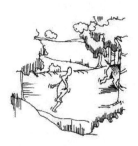

In the next picture, you see the back end of an ox running behind a big tree. Why is only the ox's rear end showing? Is the rear end the least conscious part of your dreambody? Is the ox a picture of your unconscious instincts? (Or is it the telomere, the cap on your personal history?)

For sure, your ox is a dreaming-body picture, a symbol of sensations that have gotten out of hand and are embedded behind the tree—that is, within your vegetative nervous system. For example, behind your heartbeat, or variations of that heartbeat, lies an immense power with which you may have lost contact. The same is true of all body experiences. Behind and within your symptoms, your tree, your growing and aging process, lies an immense life force. In picture 3, you have located your missing powers.

4. At last, I have my gifts in hand.

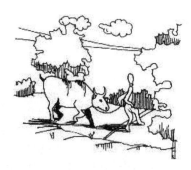

In the next picture you have found your ox and have it in hand. You tracked signals and used your attention to connect to them. Through awareness practice, here symbolized by the rope, you got a line on your power. The next task is to bring the ox home. At first the power follows your practice.

5. Oh! This "power" will not cooperate!

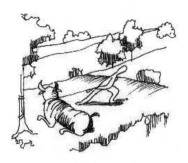

But if you thought you could easily integrate your body's power into life, you made a mistake. It does not obey your will. In this picture, you find your power now refusing to budge. It wants to remain wild, free to roam.

Zen sees this as a time that calls for the exertion of the necessary discipline to hold on to the practice. (Shamanism is similar. Don Juan tells us that we must find and then "wrestle" with our "allies," the spirits that pester us in body or mind.) You can relax only after you have found its "secret." You must be relentless in your effort to develop consistent watchfulness to transform everyday life.

Each time a symptom arises, develop the discipline of tracking and following its signals. Then hold on to your powers and find their messages, the essence behind them.

6. Ah, at last, harmony with my energy.

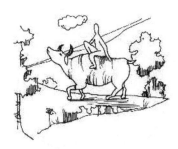

As the ox-herder, you now ride your precarious unpredictable power more steadily—that is, more coherently. This is a time of being one with your body. Both you and your ox work together, creating a kind of effortlessness. Things now happen without working on them. As you become more aligned with your power, your symptoms turn into energy for doing things.

7. What bliss!

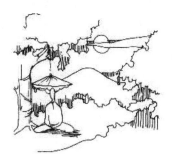

Here you feel at rest or at home in nature, sitting under a tree, quiet and peaceful. After working with your body, the sense of pain and loss of power have given way to a state of harmony with all things. Now, your body is no longer a problem for you, it is no longer on your mind or "in the picture." The ox is gone.

Things happen in nature, but you are only a witness. You are connected to the power of nature and feel restful and more secure. For many, this would be the end of focusing on their symptoms. But the reduction of symptoms through gaining access to their power was only a first step.

8. Emptiness, the force of silence.

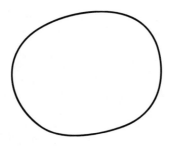

The next step is creativity. Sometimes drawings of stage 8 show nothing at all, or else a simple circle painted with one brush stroke representing the state of no-mind or emptiness that occurs. I tried to create such a spontaneous stroke with my computer.

In any case, in this state you have an empty mind, which means that you have a creative mind, open to whatever occurs. There is no painter, yet things happen. Creativity follows the force of silence. Being empty paradoxically allows you to be filled with the subtlest forces you are rarely in contact with. In this way emptiness is creativity.

9. Life . . . no body, no problem, no personal history.

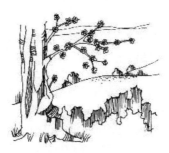

With a reduction of personal history, there is only nature, no self. In this picture, there is no you, just flowers, trees, countryside, and clouds. Your image is gone, your personal history has disappeared. As long as you had one particular identity and were possessed by constantly insisting upon your way, you marginalized your greatest power: the nonlocality of the force of silence, spread throughout the world. This power was hidden within that lost energy, that aging process, and those amplified figures in parallel universes you identified as body symptoms.

By getting closer to the powers in those symptoms, you freed yourself of your personal history and as a result became free of anxiety about your symptoms as well as about public opinion that was both for and against your old identity. Now that the world has returned in form and space and time, what about your future?

10. Back into life and the world.

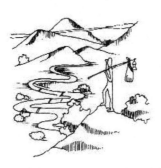

In the final picture you appear again, not quite reincarnated but seemingly thinner, having lost some weight . . . or is that weight you used to carry, now in hand, symbolized by the pack on your shoulder? In most configurations of this picture, the "you" is older, rounder, and wiser. You reenter time and the world of consensus reality that lies ahead of you in the valley.

Your path goes up and down, forward and backward, right and left without end. Your life is here symbolized by a wave, perhaps the path with heart organized by the force of silence. Now you have a lantern and a path—your awareness process and a view over the terrain. Your ordinary body is back but less prominent in the picture.

You are once again in the picture of this world, but you have changed. In a way, wherever you go and whatever you do, awareness is the point.

What this process looks like is hard to predict. When personal history is reduced, some people completely drop their old selves and open up to the world or the many worlds.

I am reminded of the words of the 104-year-old boyfriend of Amy's grandmother. He recently said to Amy and me, "The secret to my life is knowing God, trusting in God. When you are with God, you find out that you are one of God's children. If you are doubtful about things and you do not know if you are doing the right thing, talk to God and he will tell you what to do. Whatever you do is coming from God and is not you. . . . I always say, 'God, do what you want with me.' Sometimes God speaks to me and tells me to go downstairs and talk to people who seem lonely. Then they feel better. That is my work . . . now the flowers are blooming."

Exercise: Personal History As Body Experience

The following exercise explores the experience of reducing the hold of your personal history on your body. This exercise may be challenging because it will take you a bit further than you may presently be in your development. Nevertheless, I think it is important to explore where your life might be headed. The exercise gives you access to some of your power and then explores what it would be like to no longer need that power.

When you are ready, take a big breath and relax. Think back to your early childhood. Bring into your mind's eye your first childhood memory or the first intense memory of your youth. As in other exercises we have done, if you have many memories, choose one that comes to your mind first. For example, one of my readers from a minority culture in her country recalled a memory of two children playing.

Now identify two main parts, figures, or elements of this memory. Who or what was in this memory? Label these figures as "A" and "B." For example, the woman said: "A is me. B is my playmate."

Now comes a question requiring your imagination. Who or what is *left out* of this memory? What does your intuition tell you about who belongs in that memory but is not there? When you know who or what this figure or thing is, name it "C" and use a one-word description of C to represent its nature. The woman said that C was a gentle, divine, parental being. Her one-word descriptor was *parental.*

How is C's characteristic linked in some way to the history of the time in which you grew up? In what way are you and C characteristic products not only of your parents but also of the time and the nation you lived in, the race, culture, and history you are part of? The reader said that C was missing in her childhood memory of playing with her friends. In her imagination, C was a very loving person, a person very absent at that time in the history of the country she came from. No one in that country liked her people.

Choose C's strongest characteristic and ask yourself with which part of your body this characteristic is mainly associated. Feel where this characteristic may be located. What is the nature of this area? Is it symptom-free, or are there symptoms there? For example, my reader located C's parental and compassionate nature in her heart area and then realized that she suffered from pain in that area.

C is like the ox—it is something you were looking for, something hiding behind the tree in your body, perhaps in a symptom area. Now feel this body area and amplify the sense of C by focusing your breathing on that particular area. Feel C's power there. Imagine using this energy in a useful manner in your life. What good things could you do with it? How are you already using this energy in a useful way? Has it been a struggle to tame and use this energy? My reader told me that being compassionate has always been her goal. In fact, she had gone too far in being good to others and sometimes could not stop "being good-hearted," at the expense of her own needs.

Now we are going to explore reducing your personal history. Since C's characteristic is linked in part to your personal history, we are going to explore what happens when you reduce the intensity of that characteristic and the personal history associated with it.

Imagine that you have used the energy of C as much as you needed and that now its power is yours. C can become less significant. Using your breath and keeping an open mind, allow yourself to imagine reducing this characteristic, bit by bit, until it is no longer needed. At the same time, try to reduce the physical experiences you have in that body area where C is located. Notice how your body and your feelings change as you attempt to reduce this piece of your personal history.

As you reduce this body sensation and the importance of C, notice the subtle and new experiences that become available to you. What happens to your body? What feelings disappear? What new feelings arise? As you reduce this characteristic, you might notice new forms of being opening up to you. For example, my reader first resisted letting go of her compassionate nature, but then she did, and her heart area felt lighter. She realized suddenly she could be more direct with people; in fact she could even be angry, if that response arose.

Imagine living in the time and space of this new state. How could you use it in everyday life? Imagine bringing this new state into your everyday life. Who would you be? My reader was thrilled to imagine being more direct with people.

Bring this state of reduced personal history to parts of your body that are suffering or in the process of deteriorating because of aging. Make a note of your efforts.

Problems in your personal history drive you to attain certain goals, powers, and forms of behavior. This drive stresses your body because you unconsciously feel compelled to reach those goals. By discovering those powers and developing the goals of this personal history, you can eventually detach from them. That detachment reduces body stress and gives you an empty, and even more creative, mind.

Without a reduction in our personal histories, we are forever compensating for what was missing in our lives. Further, we may not only be finding but also projecting the need and tendency to reduce personal history onto our biology, onto the destruction of the DNA caps. If there is any sense at all to the biochemistry of life and aging, it is the wisdom of creating then reducing not only the genome, but personal history.

In any case, freedom from attachments to our personal history gives us the emptiness we need to get beyond, or go deeper than, even that valuable compensation. The resulting effortlessness leaves us on an unpredictable path, one in which we are moved along by the force of silence. On this path, the important thing is neither the cure of symptoms nor the achievement of worldly goals, but awareness of the journey, step by step.

18 Quantum Awareness Demons

Consciousness is part of our universe, so any physical theory which makes no proper place for it falls fundamentally short of providing a genuine description of the world. I would maintain that there is yet no physical, biological, or computational theory that comes very close to explaining our consciousness.

—*Roger Penrose, mathematician and physicist*[1]

In 1867, the Scottish physicist James Clerk Maxwell had a brainstorm and conceived of a demon that could reverse time. Until today, no one has ever been able to prove the effectiveness of his "demon" in consensus reality. It seems to me that Maxwell's demon is the projection of a more incredible kind of awareness than even Maxwell himself imagined. I suggest that his demon is a representation of awareness that operates at the immeasurable subatomic levels and is capable of upholding or at least relieving the sense of aging.

All the methods of working with symptoms that I have mentioned can be summed up under the heading of Rainbow Medicine, that is, *multileveled awareness work*. Every symptom offers a potential step toward greater awareness and creativity. In the first part of this book, I spoke of the force of silence embedded in symptoms. In part 2, you saw relationships between symptoms and community life. Until now, part 3 has focused on inner-work experiences linked to genetics, neutralizing free radicals, and relaxing cravings.

All Rainbow Medicine interventions require awareness of various dimensions and the subtle signals linked to the quantum world. In a way, each symptom is a wakeup call for lucidity and awareness. When a flickering signal becomes strong and persistent enough, you cannot pretend it is not present. Thus, Rainbow Medicine in any form is a form of awareness work.

In this chapter I discuss how increased awareness is related to increased vitality. Increasing awareness always leads to a sense of more available energy. Having more available energy is connected in physics to the second law of thermodynamics, the so-called entropy law, sometimes referred to as the "heat-death of the universe."

This law says that in all closed systems, disorder increases and the amount of available energy decreases. Another formulation of this law uses the word entropy instead of disorder. The law says that over time, entropy increases in closed systems; as they age, closed systems (described below) have less available energy for work.[2]

However, from the perspective of Rainbow Medicine, this law describes not only physical systems, but states of mind, closed and without awareness, which experience aging and fatigue. In this sense, the second law of thermodynamics can be reversed, at least at the experiential level. I will show how awareness decreases entropy, the sense of deterioration, and increases available energy. In fact, awareness may possibly reverse some forms of physical deterioration as well.

In the terms of physics, our bodies are open systems (even when we say we are closed to new ideas). Closed systems deteriorate in time. Think of a cup of black tea, just after you poured

The Entropy Law

Scientists refer to the entropy law, often called the "heat-death of the universe," as the second law of thermodynamics,[3] a universal law generally accepted by all scientists. The second law says that closed systems (such as our universe may be) will eventually deteriorate.[4]

The first law of physics is that the energy of a closed system is constant. The second law refers to available energy, which in physics means the energy that can do work. When a system is unwound, its energy may have transformed into heat, but there is none available for work.

As a student at MIT, the day I learned about that law I began wondering how to change it. I knew how it applied to our physical universe (assuming it was a closed system without consciousness), but did it apply to our bodies, symptoms, and the aging process? Let's think about entropy.

Entropy is a measure of (un)available energy but also of disorder in a system. When disorder increases, entropy increases. The second law of thermodynamics says that the CR material universe, as a closed system, moves toward disorder. According to thermodynamics, in a closed system heat, matter, and light can neither enter nor leave. Conversely, in an open system, light, heat, and matter come and go as they please.

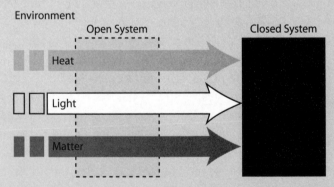

Figure 18-1. Open and Closed Systems with Heat, Light, and Matter Transfer

some milk in it, as a more-or-less closed system. At first you see the lovely design made by the milk as it swirls into the tea. But very soon, the entropy of this cup increases as that lovely design mixes in with the rest of the tea, and the order in the cup decreases. Without a fancy definition of order, let your intuition tell you what we mean by order.

The laws of nature predict that over time, the tea will become disordered. In statistical physics, there is an infinitesimal chance that the order comes back to the original design. Even, if you poured a billion cups of tea in your lifetime, such a miracle is not likely to occur.

The second law tells us just that in a closed system, the amount of information decreases as the system evolves over time. The amount of consensual information and order decrease. Note that I added the word *consensual* in the last sentence because the laws of physics concern consensual or measurable order. However, therapists know that what may be order to most people can be disorder to a particular individual.

The scientific formulation of the second law deals with the universe as a closed system (including any number of subsystems plus their environments[5]). The second law says that the entropy of a closed universe always increases; the overall amount of entropy or consensual disorder increases. Disorder increases over time. In closed systems, whatever happens leads to an increase in entropy. Formulated in terms of order, the second law of thermodynamics says that in a universe (or any closed system), the net amount of order cannot increase but must decrease. Known patterns go to pieces!

Everything inside of you may rebel against this law, and indeed, since Rudolf Clausius originally formulated this second law, many scientists have rebelled. However, to date, no one has been able to defy this law. Deterioration and aging happen to all closed universes. In some ways, the second law seems like common sense. If you leave a damp car inside a closed garage, 100 years later the car will be rusted to pieces. That is a mundane example of the second law of thermodynamics.

Nevertheless, there is always a rebel who refuses to concede the truth of this law. "There *must be* local and temporary order;

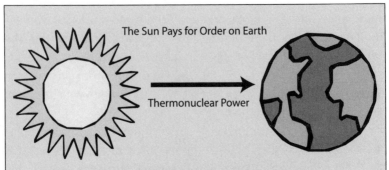

The Sun Pays for Order on Earth

Thermonuclear Power

Figure 18-2. The Earth's Order Costs the Sun's Dis-Order

Because the Earth is an open system penetrated by the radiant heat energy of the sun (as well as energy from the rest of the universe), to increase its own order, the Earth uses the sun's energy. If we pretend for the moment that the Earth and sun are a closed system, the second law says that order on the Earth results in the sun burning out. Our evolution, development, creative ideas, and new tools are all based upon decreasing the thermonuclear power of the sun. We are only an enclave of order. Using less fuel and buying fewer things only puts off the inevitable heat-death of the sun and eventually the Earth. Our momentary life is linked to the sun's death.

after all, life is orderly and meaningful. The human race is an example of increasing order. Evolution creates order. Even Darwin said we are evolving."

But physicists respond, "No! The local order is only temporary. Disorder in the rest of the disorderly universe pays for local order on Earth. You and I and the rest of the human race, our evolution and that of other species, are all examples of open systems living on a planet basking in the sun. Momentary order is paid for at the expense of the sun!"

Does the Entropy Law Apply to People?

Yes, of course it does. We, along with everything else in a closed system, are likely to degenerate eventually in terms of CR measures of energy and the capacity to do work. Even as open systems that eat and take in things from the outside world, we tend to degenerate slowly over the decades.

However, if awareness is present, Maxwell's fantasy of a demon who reverses the second law (see next section) may have been right. The next exercise shows that the amount of energy you feel is available to you at any given moment depends upon your level of awareness. In other words, the second law is correct for all closed material and psychological systems without awareness. All the laws of physics are patterns of our universe—devoid of awareness.

Consider closed and open systems. We often speak of people as being "open" or "closed," referring to their personalities. In both physics and psychology, closed systems are systems—people or things—who are inflexible and unable or unwilling to take in new stuff from the outside. The entropy law in physics describes a consensus reality universe that is impervious. Whether or not new concepts of gravity or parallel universes will eventually change this view remains to be seen. But in the moment, in its present form, physics describes a universe whose loss of information—a kind of unconsciousness, in psychological terms—increases over time. Unconsciousness eventually leads to lack of awareness of who and where you are, and where your process is going.

The Maxwell Demon— A Quantum Demon

James Clerk Maxwell's brainstorm in 1867, in which he conceived of a force that could reverse time, described an awareness demon that could reverse the entropy law by tracking the tiny movements of molecules in a gas. In this way, the demon could reverse the disorder in closed systems, at least in his fantasy.

Maxwell's imaginary demon sat in a closed box and reversed the flow of molecules to recreate order that was degenerating.[6] The demon, a prototype of consciousness in matter, noticed things happening and controlled them by making special choices.

He kept hot stuff on one side of the box and cooler stuff on the other side, so that the original order (of hot and cold) would not deteriorate. The demon set things up so that energy does not have to become less available and information does not have to be lost in a closed system. By using awareness to open and shut partitions dividing two volumes of a gas in a container, the demon reversed the second law. To date, no one has yet found such a demon or been able to produce one in consensus reality.

Yet, Maxwell's fantasy may be more correct than he realized. It seems to me that he may have been projecting our capacity for lucidity, our ability to notice nano-events or flirts. This almost immeasurable quantum awareness is an awareness ability that can make choices in dreamland.

Maxwell's demon is the potential hero of psychotherapy, for it is the part of us that reverses messes by seeing patterns where old ones were lost (forgotten, repressed, ignored, marginalized). To me, the second law of thermodynamics is a projection of the typical CR lifestyle that uses minimal awareness. Maxwell's demon is a representation of our lucid awareness that operates at the immeasurable subatomic levels of nano-like events and which is capable of at least relieving the sense of aging.

The psychological principle projected onto Maxwell's demon is this: Seeing the order hidden in CR disorder creates more available energy.

Ignoring or even repressing subtle signals of symptoms is depressing and exhausting. Recognizing symptoms as wake-up calls for attention allows you to make order out of disorder and gives you generally more available energy with which to work. Marginalizing experience makes you feel like a rundown universe.

I call Maxwell's demon a quantum awareness demon, a lucid ray of consciousness that tracks the motions of atoms and molecules as well as subatomic events. Quantum mechanics was not yet invented during Maxwell's life. He did not yet know about wave functions; that theory would come 50 years later. But if he lived today, he would surely have been interested in the kind of awareness that was capable of noticing and tracking subtle tendencies, dreamland quantum waves, and the guidance they give us. In my imagination he would have said that ignoring all the subtle feelings that flicker in our awareness contributes to exhaustion and makes us feel older than we are.

Exercise: Neg-Entropy Awareness

The following exercise gives you a chance to discover and test this demon's ability to increase the amount of physical energy available to you. We will focus especially on closed areas of your life.

Make yourself comfortable and consider how you feel about aging. What do you like about it? What don't you like about it? For example, many people love the chance of growing into their potential but dislike the loss of energy and what they call good looks. Some have the idea that life is going to end.

When you are ready, look around for something to lift or push. If you are standing in a room, lift a chair or push against one of the walls and see how much available energy you have. While lifting or pushing, ask yourself, "What percentage of my energy is available right now?" Make a note of the amount of energy now. Is it 85 percent or 50 percent or 15 percent? How old do you feel? For example, when I lift a chair today, it feels heavier than it ought to. I'd say, 50 percent of my energy is available to me.

The amount of available or isometric energy that you have depends very much on your sense of order inside yourself. So now think of one area of your life that feels disorderly. If possible, choose a new area, not relationships or body symptoms, since we have worked on those before. For example, your work, your finances, perhaps the mess on your desk, or the way you use time seems disorderly. Perhaps the way you deal with criticism is disorderly.

Don't overlook ignored areas of your life in need of order. If there are many areas, choose just one for the moment, any one will do. How do you manage to avoid this area? In what sense is this area closed? Do you forget or avoid the issues associated with this area? How do you forget these issues? Do you try to sleep more? Do you just complain about them? Do you push them out of your mind? Do you watch TV or go to the movies instead of cleaning up this area?

Now while thinking of that disorderly area, imagine the kind of space it is in. What colors and motions take place in that space? Use your own words to describe the characteristics of the space containing this disordered area of life. For example, is it gray or muddy? Is it swirling and mixed-up?

If you could identify a location outside your body where this disorderly area might be, where would that space be located? (e.g., in front of you, behind you, etc.) Sketch that disorderly area near your body. How does the part of your body closest to this space feel? Do you have symptoms in your body near that area? Choose a body symptom, or one of those symptoms, to work on, perhaps the one that has received the least attention from you. Is that symptom possibly connected with your sense of aging?

Focus on a symptom in that area of the body and identify two of its aspects. For example, see if you can form an image of the energy you suspect/imagine to be causing that symptom, and then do the same for the receiver of that energy or action. In other words, imagine a "symptom maker" and a "symptom receiver."

One way to imagine these two figures is to feel into, or imagine feeling into the symptom as much as is possible. Then exaggerate that feeling, amplifying its intensity. Using your attention, stay with that feeling until a figure emerges that might embody such intensity. For example, if you have a pounding headache, you might exaggerate the feeling of that pounding until an angry figure emerges, banging on a table, and a sensitive figure emerges (perhaps the table itself), hurt by the pounding.

Try to find out the message that each figure is expressing. For example, the angry figure might be saying, "I have to pound my way through things," while the other says, "Please don't do things that way, it is just too harsh, and it hurts me!"

Imagine the two figures, the one suffering and the other creating the symptom. Even sketch them. Then allow your imagination to spontaneously create a being whose awareness enters the field and resolves the conflict between those two energies. Perhaps imagine a master facilitator, a genie, a spirit, a cartoon character—something that can deal with the two energies. Describe it. Draw it.

One of my readers had a conflict between her worldly ambitiousness and the part of her that was weighed down by the pressure of that ambition. To her surprise, she saw a priest who helped her facilitate a resolution of the conflict between these two energies. The priest blessed both parts of her, and both relaxed.

At some point, you might try to become your helpful spirit, your quantum awareness demon. Step into the psychologically closed system of your dreaming body and intervene; facilitate the conflict between the two parts in that symptom area.

Imagine the resulting story. Allow the quantum demon to intervene in a magical way and find a resolution. The reader with the ambitiousness in her symptoms found, to her surprise, that both conflicting parts missed God, represented by the priest. At first this reader was shy about identifying with the priest, until she realized that in some ways, she had already devoted her life to "divine things."

Use your breathing to focus on the feeling of that resolution. If possible, feel a sense of resolution in that symptom area.

Imagine how this resolution might be used in the disordered area of life with which you began this exercise. Recall the original mess—its space, colors, and motions—and notice (better yet, even draw) how that area has transformed. Don't "work" at this, just let things happen inside until resolutions occur.

Finally, go back to the wall or chair and, being careful, again see the effect this work may have had on your sense of available energy to do what you need to do in life. What changes in your available energy do you notice?

Quantum Awareness Demons

There were several goals in this exercise. One was to notice the messes in your life and realize how they affect or relate to your body. Another was to learn that whenever your energy feels drained, you may be tired, but you may also be suffering from too much entropy—disorder and lost energy.

Disordered areas are like closed systems, ruled by the unconsciousness of conflicts. Bringing awareness to these areas reverses your sense of aging by giving you more available energy. Your sense of the forward march of time is accentuated by inner conflicts that are being ignored or closed off. By using awareness, conflicting energies in that messy area become more coherent with one another. Instead of working *with* yourself, you were working against yourself. Focusing awareness on internal conflicts increases your sense of wellness by reversing the conflict and increasing your internal coherence.

Every mess reflects your choice to ignore your awareness potential. In the ordinary world, you may feel like you are aging rapidly or are physically weak because of inner conflicts and unavoidable deterioration. However, access to your awareness may reverse this feeling by creating more order and available energy and a resulting sense of wellness.[7]

Every area of disorder is like a symptom: There are two energies in conflict, and no resolving essence. The result is a situation where you have two "horses" pulling against each other instead of together. Without awareness, you call this submerged conflict situation fatigue and aging. With awareness, you add a hyperspace and reverse the direction of time. Get to know that awareness demon from another realm for whom no CR system is permanently closed.

19 Death, the End?

Nothing in life is to be feared. It is only to be understood.

—*Marie Curie*[1]

To consider that after the death of the body the spirit perishes is like imagining that a bird in a cage will be destroyed if the cage is broken, though the bird has nothing to fear from the destruction of the cage.

Our body is like the cage, and the spirit like the bird. We see that without the cage this bird flies in the world of sleep; therefore, if the cage becomes broken, the bird will continue and exist. Its feelings will be even more powerful, its perceptions greater, and its happiness increased.

—*Abdu'l-Baha*[2]

For some, it's a relief when death knocks on the door. Something deep inside says, "Happy day; free of myself and my limitations!" But death is full of paradoxes. On the one hand, when you first realize you are actually dying, you usually fear it. Perhaps you don't tell your friends initially because telling them would mean more trouble. Like you, they live in the world of consensus reality and focus only upon the eventual loss of the physical form.

For your CR mind and your friends, death is usually a robbery, not a gift. Yet if you think about it, for the person who is dying, death can spell freedom from everything, including the concept of death itself, at least death as "the end." Near death, the dreams you have will probably be about going on with life. Seemingly ignoring the idea of an end, many people dream about their next steps, often into well-known hyperspaces. Some dream of studying in "classes" unlike any known on Earth; others dream of becoming birds that fly in the dream as if they had been birds their whole lives.

In this book I have considered the disorders of life to be problems to work through, to be areas of life hiding other worlds and new kinds of order and meaning. But now I want to look at disorder in a new way, as if the process of apparent chaos itself were meaningful. What seems like death's "disordering" process is only the end of your identity in CR. No longer do you have a single disorder—a kidney or heart problem, a lung or stomach illness, or an ovary, breast, or prostate tumor. Now the whole body is a huge disorder. Aging leads to increased entropy in your physical body, but in dreamland, this isn't the end. Death is often reinterpreted in dreams as the path of freedom from the old self. New things are now possible.

Phases of Dying

There are many phases to death. The threat of death at first comes like the scolding of a schoolteacher. Get your life together! After fighting like a school kid, you try to complete what you feel is most meaningful. Death says, "Stop hesitating in relationships. Go for your grandest visions, become your whole self." Perhaps you have stood at many edges in your life and hesitated instead of moving forward. Now death gives you a needed push.

At another point the threat of death becomes the threat of a full-blown version of an altered (foggy or quiet) state that seems to be only in its beginning stages. In a way, the full-blown state is trying to happen right now, refusing to wait until the end of your life. Death as an altered state threatens to become a part of this life, not just because death is approaching, but because you are too one-sided in your lifestyle, too clear, too extroverted, too interested in what people think. Experiencing everyday life without the simultaneous and parallel awareness of the existence of death's altered states is like standing in the sun without casting a shadow on the ground.

"Death is your greatest ally," claims the shaman don Juan. A quantum physicist interested in parallel worlds would say, emphatically, there is no death without life.[3] In what Rainbow Medicine calls dreamland and physics calls the mathematics of physics, life and death are both simultaneously present (in parallel worlds). Nothing can be alive if it is not also dead, and nothing can be dead in CR if it has no life in dreamland. The imminence of CR death opens up awareness to the dreamland hyperspaces in everyday life. Added to life, death creates fantasy and detachment.

In still another phase of the dying process, death becomes the threat of extreme altered states of consciousness. Death challenges you to develop your ability to navigate through the visions and pains typified by the *bardos* (otherworldly states or realms) in the Tibetan Book of the Dead. In these altered states, many people briefly meet the unresolved problems in life, cravings they never satisfied, and that old rigid personality again, this time as a gruesome mask, perhaps. At this stage of life, the threat of death invites you to become acquainted with the quantum world of visions, the dreamworld of monsters and bardos.[4] In my limited experience, these visions pass quickly or may not appear, especially if you have wrestled with some of these monsters earlier in life.

In life, death is a strict Zen master, an awareness teacher standing in front of you with a stick. Without awareness, painkillers and morphine may be the best option through these difficult bardo states of wonder and trouble. I don't blame anyone who wants to spend their last days drugged. However, from the experiences I have had working with people near death, it seems to me that nothing more wonderful could happen than to develop your familiarity with meditation and fantasy techniques that enable you to experience some of the most awesome states at the end of your life. If you learn how to deal with altered states of consciousness, life near death may seem like a wonder.[5]

When death comes knocking on the door, there is no longer any desire for CR "healings" for that old body. People who fight death too long can avoid becoming lucid about their inner truth and most authentic pattern. Those who can open up to deathlike events find not meaninglessness, but an old friend close to chaos. The Sufi poet Rumi formulated this idea in the twelfth century when he wrote:

> If you can't do this work yourself, don't worry.
> You don't even have to make a decision, one way or another.
> The Friend, who knows a lot more than you do,
> will bring difficulties, and grief, and sickness,
> as medicine, as happiness,
> as the essence of the moment you are beaten
> when you hear checkmate,
> and can finally say with Allah's voice,
> I trust you to kill me.[6]

To see what happens when your everyday mind surrenders, I have devised two exercises. The first deals with creativity, and the second with navigating comatose states.

Chaos and Creativity

To understand something about the fearsome chaos and creativity in near-death experiences and to prepare for such states,

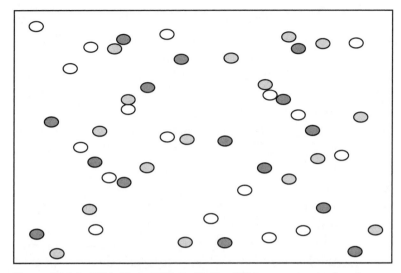

Figure 19-1. Let This Picture Flirt with You. When you are ready, relax your eyes, take a deep breath, and "let go." Feel as dreamy as you can and let the picture flirt with you—that is, take your time and let something quickly catch your attention, something irrational. Hold that in your memory. What caught your attention?

take a look at figure 19-1. Let's experiment with your awareness process using this picture. Are you ready? Read what is written under the picture.

At first, most people can't make out anything in that picture and are uncomfortable with its chaos. Then, with patience, most people see all sorts of things flickering with their attention. For example, some people see symmetrical stars or an image of the universe; others see empty space, musical notes, rain and sunshine, swarms of butterflies, and wrapping paper. Someone even saw a stop sign!

If you did this experiment, it may have shown you that if you relax and accept chaos, if you surrender, the force of silence inevitably creates new things. The point is that what appears as chaos and disorder in one world is a pattern filled with potential information in another. In death, or near death, when chaotic states of disorder break down our consensual order, a new universe and way of life often can emerge. *Life* does not refer only to

the existence of the physical body; it also includes the spontaneity and creativity of awareness. Dreaming recreates the universe.[7]

The concept of death can be scary, but when it opens you up,
old identities fall away and the possibility of change arises. This
reminds me of the last words of Peter, with whom Amy and I
worked some years ago, a courageous man who was dying from
leukemia. With our help, he came out of a coma and temporarily
back to life before quietly dying. Before he died he shouted,
yelling ecstatically in his hospital room in Zurich, "I . . . have . . .
found . . . it. I . . . have . . . found . . . the . . . thing . . . I . . . have
always looked for. The . . . key . . . to . . . life . . . the key is a new
tram . . . plan . . . everything is in the plan. . . . Everything . . . it
. . . was here . . . even before you began to work with me."[8]

Until the last stage of his life, Peter worked for the popular
Zurich newspaper, the *Tages Anzeiger,* writing about the news in
Switzerland. We could say that only in consensus reality was he a
real person. The plan that appeared just then, at the end of his
life, was a kind of pilot wave—a map of the city tram system with
its multiple tracks through Zurich. His intentional wave was a new
map for Zurich. He realized that his particular form of interconnectedness was simultaneously the structure of a "new" Zurich.

From the largest viewpoint, we are all maps; we are all composed of the lines of intentional fields experienced physically as
the force of silence. When disorder becomes inevitable through
the experience of illness, loss, or upheaval of some sort, it disrupts
your consensual path. Yet an ordered plan, which was always
there, can reappear. If we relax our CR identity as a person
located in a body, our real selves appear as a kind of immortal
intent, a nonlocal plan spread everywhere and including everyone
whose intent is similar.

The Nobel Prize-winning physicist Wolfgang Pauli must have
realized this too, because he said, just before he died, "Dreaming
is the background of physics." Earlier I quoted an Australian
Aboriginal saying, "You can kill the kangaroo, but you can't kill the
kangaroo dreaming." I mentioned Lewis O'Brien, the Aboriginal
elder who showed how the street plan of the city of Adelaide was

built on the outline of the Red Kangaroo, without anyone having realized this.[9] Our immortal, timeless pattern is an aspect of the Earth's or universe's structure.

Comatose States

At various times in my life I have been scared of dying. Now, after having worked with many people going through altered states while they were dying, I feel relieved. Comatose states near death inevitably seem to reveal important directions, new phases, plans, and maps that manifest the intentional field more palpably than anywhere else in life.[10]

Deterioration and chaos are not the only rulers of comatose-like states that occur near death. Coma is not the end of awareness. If we judge from the experiences of people who have gone through comatose experiences, and also from stories and recorded facts from Tibetan masters who "died" in Western hospitals and still maintained unusual body heat days after "death,"[11] we must consider the possibility of awareness continuing after apparent death.

Today's diagnosis of death, based on unresponsiveness of the brain or spinal cord, will soon be insufficient. As nanoscience develops, responsiveness will be measured at the atomic level, which will complicate today's CR definitions of death. Life will be measured in terms of nano-responses.

Experimenting with strongly altered or comatose states of consciousness is one of the simplest, yet most dramatic, ways of finding the force of silence. The following material may help you work with yourself and others in these near-death states.[12] The work involves a combination of using your lucid attention to follow CR signals (such as breathing, slight movements of the hand and eyelid) as well as subtle, nonconsensual signals (such as flirts, visions, or intuitions). Awareness at all levels is the key. To explore the potential creativity inherent in near-death states, remember the Maxwell demon. Use your imagination in coma-like states.

Exercise: Coma—
the Moment of Awakening

To begin, relax for a few minutes, noticing the rhythmic inflow and outflow of your breathing, letting that rhythm lull you into a drifting, comfortable state. When you feel ready, imagine that you just drift off into a comatose state. Take your time with this imaginary experience. As you are drifting off, you may realize that some of your fatigue states were attempts to get to this altered state of consciousness. While relaxed and in a coma-like state, just follow your own breathing in this state, being aware only of your breath.

Use your relaxed but lucid attention. After a while, when something catches your attention, perhaps a body twitch or jitter, notice and follow that experience. Use your lucidity and trust in your tiny experiences. Above all, catch little awakening tendencies. For example, your eyelids may begin to open spontaneously on their own, or your fingers or hands move on their own. Perhaps a sound caught your attention. Notice the moment when some sound or movement tendency occurs.

This is a very creative moment. After catching it, take a few minutes and marvel at the spontaneous nature of the force of your dreaming and, using the rhythm of your breath, let it unfold. Perhaps visions, fantasies, even stories emerge. Be a witness to your own experience, even if it seems very irrational at first.

When your fantasy has had time to emerge and complete itself, you may find yourself feeling more awake and wanting to move. In this case it's time to wonder about the significance of your fantasy and experience. Might life's path be embedded or symbolized in this fantasy? For example, a shy, elderly woman who was afraid of dying did this exercise and experienced what she called a bird awakening her. As she lay quietly in her garden, doing this exercise, the sound of one of the birds snapped her gently out of her state. At first she could hardly believe in the significance of those birds, because they had frequently caught her attention. But now she let her fantasy unfold and found herself flying around freely, like a bird, looking over the houses of her family, giving them advice. "What a surprise," she told me, "to discover that giving advice is so central to me." After this experience, she dropped her shyness and allowed her family to benefit more from her wisdom.

This exercise may have given you a sense not only of near-death experiences but also of the spontaneous energies and creativity that appear when your CR focus is reduced. Then the force of silence can be heard best, and you realize that it is always there. Perhaps you went so deeply that you discovered a part of a larger and more basic pattern characterizing your life. Such patterns may be the corollary of what quantum physicists such as Werner Heisenberg call the tendencies of quantum waves—predispositions of CR reality.

The Timeless Path

In my experience, the sensations and events that occur in reduced states of consciousness, such as may have occurred for you in the previous exercise, are typical of near-death states even though our physiology while doing it is very different near death. Such experiences of buried maps and flying like a bird may encourage you to consider new parts of yourself that make you into a new kind of person—a person with a multileveled awareness that has more facets of global and hyperspatial perspectives. The person emerging from near-death experiences always seems to me to be more human and conscious, capable of identifying with infinity and, at the same time, with the human species and all planetary life.

This new person is on the path behind all paths. This path is likely behind all you do and have done, as well as all you dreamed you could have done. Just as the pilot wave is the sum of all the parallel worlds in which it may manifest, all possible paths you take are different tributaries of the more central, timeless path.

For example, one of your parallel worlds or paths may be your CR identity, your everyday self. Another path includes the people you love the most; on another path are the people you detest. Still others may include thieves, healers, lovers, and enemies, ambition, generosity, even death.

In quantum theory, a particle can be understood as simultaneously taking each of its possible paths. Likewise, in dreams you may find yourself taking all these paths in a given night, even though you tend to choose one of these paths at a time in everyday reality.

Carlos Castaneda describes his awesome shamanic teacher, don Juan Matus, in *Journey to Ixtlan*. Speaking of all paths, don Juan said that "each path is only a path." From don Juan's essence perspective, all paths go nowhere. Since each path is only a path, the wise person chooses the special path with heart, which is free of fear and ambition. This is the path you choose as a very old or wise person. This timeless path makes you feel well and joyful. It is the sum and the essence of all the other paths, the one that appears most clearly near the end of your CR life or in deep altered states.

Aboriginal belief understands the relationship between the various worlds of reality and dreaming as the two faces of the moon. The light part represents everyday reality, whereas the dark part is the dreaming, that part of the moon you do not see when you observe its bright face on a moonlit night.[13] In a way, the dark side of the moon is another image of the force behind dreaming, the force of silence. Even when the bright side of the moon is not visible, the dark side is there, preparing for a renewal of the light. Order and disorder are both part of our human pattern, as they are part of the pattern of the universe.

I was recently amazed to discover that similar ideas about the moon are also found in Taoism. According to sinologist Dr. Frank Fiedeler, "The concept of change [named in *The Book of Changes* or *I Ching*] was originally based on the changes of light and darkness in the phases of the moon. In its most ancient form, the Chinese character *yi*, meaning 'change,' was a pictograph showing the moon's dark and bright sides."[14]

Apparently symbolizing the dark and light sides of the moon, the pictograph *yi* represents the changes of the moon. The basic idea is that as one part of life becomes visible, invisibility declines, and vice versa. As something becomes conscious, the unknown declines.

This way of thinking is richly represented in the enigmatic and mysterious ancient sayings of the Chinese *I Ching*, which attempts to explain the principles of change. According to the *I Ching*, "Counting that which is going into the past depends on the forward movement. Knowing that which is to come depends on the backward movement. This is why the *Book of Changes* has backward moving numbers."[15]

In the *Tao Te Ching*, the legendary founder of Taoism, Lao Tse, says that the "Tao which can be said is not the eternal Tao." In this statement, Lao Tse is placing the emphasis in life not upon the visible but upon the invisible—motivations or tendencies behind things. The physicist David Bohm said something very similar about the wave function as a universal but invisible flux behind things: ". . . there is a universal flux that cannot be defined explicitly but which can be known only implicitly, as indicated by the explicitly definable forms and shapes, some stable and some unstable, that can be abstracted from the universal flux. In this flow, mind and matter are not separate substances. Rather, they are different aspects of one whole and unbroken movement."[16]

Beyond Zero-Sum Games

The force of silence, the path with heart, the Tao which cannot be said, the *Tai Chi*, the dreaming, Bohm's pilot wave—all are aspects of a basic pattern behind what we consider in everyday reality to be our psychophysical nature. In everyday life, you easily neglect this path that produces the ups and down, the balance in life. Neglecting this path makes us fear death, in part to find the timeless way. This subtle path cannot be measured or calculated; in a way, it is "nothing" from a CR perspective. Yet because of its nonlocality and timelessness, it is a central or essential life experience. Without it, life is depressingly one-dimensional.

In the 1930s, a prominent mathematical physicist of the time, John von Neumann, the man who first clarified the math behind quantum physics, showed how math came from the mind. Mind was the primal reality giving rise to math, and from math came the physical world. The idea was that the CR physical world was a manifestation of math (such as quantum wave function). In other words, the CR world was a manifestation of deeper realities, and not the fundamental reality.

Everyday reality by itself is depressing because it is a kind of "zero-sum game," to use a von Neumann term. There is only so much life to be had in CR. Whatever you do, you are not likely at this point in history to increase your life span much beyond 120 years. You can't beat death.

Under these circumstances, you can make a choice: Stay in the CR game or shift to a more primal reality, your awareness of the force of silence. Coming from another time and space, this nonlocal pattern manifests in the tiniest, micro-physiological movements and in apparently insignificant flirt-like ideas. Notice these tendencies, live closer to this prime reality, the intent which moves beyond your individual lifetime. This intent is beyond time. Then you know that CR concepts such as time and space, life and death, person and particle are insufficient to describe the timeless spaceless path you have been on—and may always be on.

IV
QUANTUM DEMON LIFESTYLES: THE BODY FREE OF TIME

20 Nonlocal Medicine in Practice

Quantum systems have internal relationships.
After meeting, each becomes part of something
new which is larger than itself.
                                        —Dona Zohar[1]

To the enlightened man . . . whose consciousness embraces the universe, to him the universe
becomes his "body," while the physical body
becomes a manifestation of the Universal Mind.
                                        —Lama Anagarika[2]

We have seen that Maxwell's demon is a projection of the
kind of awareness that reverses disorder by being awake even
in chaotic states and near-death situations. The second law of
thermodynamics turns out to be the fairy tale of what happens

when "no one is home"—when there is no awareness in the closed system. This "law" is a projection of the typical modern lifestyle that uses minimal awareness and, as a result, is always uncertain where the available energy comes from or goes to. Maxwell's demon reverses all that by bringing light to a dark home, bringing lucidity to immeasurable, nano-like events—a lucidity that finds available energy just about anywhere. In the last part of the book, I suggest ways to integrate this lucidity into daily life.

In Rainbow Medicine, the concept of the person is like the concept of a particle in physics. Just as point particles don't exist in consensus reality, neither do specific entities called people. At essence, we are fields described by the force of silence moving us along its path, spread out everywhere our intent is shared.

Nonlocality plays a central role in life and therefore in Rainbow Medicine concepts and practice. Like all events, symptoms are not located *only* in the physical body. Although appearing mainly as observable characteristics requiring local body treatments, symptoms also have nonconsensual, space-like positions requiring treatment where they appear—in relationships, community, the world, the past, and the future.

While most modern medical scientists consider healing an essentially local phenomenon connected to the patient's body, shamans have always been more community-oriented. Shamans have employed the underlying phenomenon of nonlocality for centuries to help people at a distance. I suspect that a deeper understanding of nonlocal medicine and its effects will change the practice of medicine by more completely incorporating the experiences of the community—and of course the doctor—into the health condition of the patient. Today, most doctors are trained to shut down their feelings, to keep their emotions separate from their interactions with their patients.

Theoretically and experientially, you and I are bathed in dreamlike fields that make symptom work local, nonlocal—and fantastic. Without this larger perspective, we are forced to practice

Process-Oriented Medicine Concepts

INTENTIONAL OR PILOT WAVES: Pilot waves are a Bohmian concept derived from the quantum wave function. The field of such waves is experienced as subtle tendencies or the force of silence. These waves and this force are information experienced as guidance. Their intent is never clearly known until experiences unfold themselves.

THE QUANTUM DEMON OF AWARENESS: The Maxwellian demon is a projection of consciousness or awareness onto matter, a projection of the human and universe's tendency toward self-reflection. In your personal life, quantum awareness demons appear in your exquisite ability to notice and return flirts. Though most physicists think quantum events are virtual realities that are closed off to everyday awareness, the demon's lucid awareness cracks open the apparently sealed-off nature of the CR world and senses tendencies and the force of silence beyond what is measured or predictable in CR (according to the second law of thermodynamics).

In other words, to the everyday mind, awareness only appears to be closed off from subtle, nano-type events. But like Maxwell's demon, awareness can reverse everyday common events. The demon cannot be discovered in consensus reality, not because it does not exist, but because it may reside in the reflecting ability of immeasurable quantum events. In quantum theory we find it in the math.[3] In you and me, the demon appears in our awareness of flirts. The demon is everyone's natural inheritance, the lucid ability found everywhere in nature's self-reflections, which give rise to a real world of appearances. That demon can track the subtlest force of silence, and it remains conscious even when the everyday mind is asleep.

The demon's self-reflecting tendencies create the probabilities of existence and life. It is a personification of the ability of the force of silence to self-reflect.

OBSERVATION AND MARGINALIZATION: Self-reflecting tendencies in the force of silence create CR reality. In turn, our awareness can marginalize parallel worlds and the force of silence as if they did not exist. Ignoring imaginary qualities of life allows us to create a consensual everyday reality focused mostly upon measurable objects and ideas. Marginalized realities reappear imbedded in things we call problems, people, and symptoms.

NONLOCALITY: Nonlocality is the spaceless and timeless quality of tendencies. (In the math of physics, and in your inner experience, nonlocality can have a space-like and time-like quality.) Nonlocal information manifests in dreams, fantasies, intuitions, vague fields, and entangling flirts—bits and short-lived pieces of consensus reality (too rapid, unrepeatable, or irrational to measure).

UNFOLDING AND SUPERPOSITION: The force of silence self-reflects, unfolds, and manifests in CR reality via a multitude of dream-like fragments and fleeting observations scattered throughout the day and night. These fragments and observations remain essentially separate from consensus reality; they exist in parallel worlds, as if they were separate universes. Superposition means that each and every fragment is part of the sum of what I refer to metaphorically as the path with heart. Each separate world is a face of the force of silence.

some form of one-dimensional local medicine, while splitting off the vivid experiences and projections that connect us in a multidimensional universe.

Communication and Parallel Worlds

Before exploring how to use the nonlocality of the relationship between "doctor and patient" as a form of medicine, I summarize ideas from this book that are necessary for what comes next.

Nonlocality describes many of the subtle feelings of interconnectedness we have with all beings. Rainbow Medicine engages nonlocal realities in various ways to work with symptoms. For example, in previous chapters I have pointed out nonlocal connections between your body symptoms, your personal relationships, and your community problems. Now I want to explore nonlocal worlds of relationships available when working with symptoms.

Like all other events, communication between human beings is multileveled. Each signal exchange involves multiple realities. In the first place, we send one another CR signals with which we can identify; that is, we communicate in a way that can be heard and seen. What we say and do can be picked up with a video camera.

Signals and Double Signals

As an example of signals and double signals, imagine your client tells you she is worried about something. In response, you reply, "Don't worry."

What you don't quite notice, however, is that your client is also saying, with her head tilted downward and a downtrodden expression on her face, "I am depressed." You notice her signs on a video but did not see them when speaking with her. On the video you also notice that your shoulders suddenly hunch up, as if to say, "I don't know what to do," in response to her downtrodden expression. The following diagram sketches these two sets of dynamics.

CR signals are intended and their existence will be agreed upon, whereas double signals are not intended, and a common meaning is, without awareness, difficult to notice and agree upon. (For example, we have all learned to smile at one another, while ignoring other, subtler double signals.)

As the lower half of the picture implies, our double signals are entangled with one another. Unintentional signals elicit subtle responses of discomfort or unease that may be unfolded, with the use of awareness, into communicated feelings such as "I don't know what to do," "I will help!" or "I don't care!" We cannot

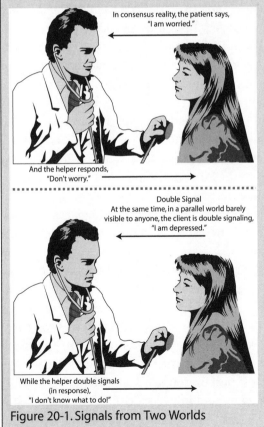

In consensus reality, the patient says, "I am worried."

And the helper responds, "Don't worry."

Double Signal
At the same time, in a parallel world barely visible to anyone, the client is double signaling, "I am depressed."

While the helper double signals (in response), "I don't know what to do!"

Figure 20-1. Signals from Two Worlds

always easily identify who did what first by studying that video of double signals. Like all dreamland events, your and your client's signals are nonlocal, that is, they are interconnected, entangled processes.

In addition to visible signals and double signals that can be seen with a video camera, let's not forget those pre-signals that you feel and sense, but which do not yet appear on the surface of CR reality. Pre-signals are often flirt-like body experiences, too subtle to be seen on a video, though they do appear to our lucid awareness as flirts and flashes. In time, they usually express themselves as visible signals.

We identify with some of these visible CR signals, whereas we seem to be unconscious of the other visible signals we are sending.

I call signals we send (and can be seen on a video camera), but do not identify with secondary or double signals. We do not realize we are sending them.[4] I found that the messages in these signals can be seen in dreams. For example, you may be unaware of being excited and sending out enthusiastic signals, and dream of enthusiastic dreamfigures.

Double dreamland signals and the subtle flirts and deep essence feelings entangle us with one another, making a relationship a multidimensional and amazing event. Relationship could be defined as the sum of your CR relationship identities (e.g., doctor-patient, student-student, parent-child, friend-friend, lovers, etc.) plus all the intertwined dreamland and essence signals and experiences. The CR you and I are just two facets of the force of silence in our relationship.

The essence and dreamland worlds are basically nonlocal. Their signals and pre-signals are difficult to clearly locate as originating in either you or me. They are everywhere. Yet all these separate and often conflicting sets of signals (such as saying yes, while unwittingly shaking the head no) contribute to the many worlds and relationships we share with one another. What we call relationship is really a superposition, a composition of all worlds, most of which are marginalized in everyday life. For example, in one world we agree; in another, we may be in the middle of an argument. In one world you may be the doctor and I the patient; however, in another world, you may be a child while I am a parent.

We are always involved in multiple roles in relationships. Each role combination is a whole world! For example, in addition to helper and client, in all relationships you will find some of the following dual roles: friend-friend, guru-disciple, parent-child, abuser-abused, teacher-student, employer-employee, female-male, gay-gay, etc. Again, what we call relationship is an unbelievable rainbow of colors, a virtual superposition of all these roles or worlds. If there is a conflict in a marginalized, unrecognized world, the CR relationship is in trouble! Lucidity of subtle flirts and general awareness of all kinds of signals and pre-signals are needed in everyday life to resolve unacknowledged issues that can be seen only in dreams.

Relationship Ethics

What do multidimensional rainbow concepts intersect with in everyday practice? How do you deal with all these roles once you know about them? I use the following guidelines for clarity in my work.[5]

• *Respect.* Respect the identified and preferred CR relationship. If you contract with someone to be in the role of a helper, then make that your main focus. Inquire about and respect the other's needs.

• *Sharing roles.* Since all the other possible roles are needed to be a helper, bring them into your awareness and share them— with the interest and agreement of the person seeking help. If you do not receive consent to share your awareness of these other roles, use your insights for your own life. (How to do so will be clearer after the examples below.)

• *Power differences.* Seen from the viewpoint of a given social reality, each relationship involves power differences, such as that between parent and child, student and teacher, doctor and patient, even two friends (one is more dominant than the other). These differences must be made explicit to avoid fearful, hurtful, or defensive body reactions.

For example, if you are feeling like a child when a client arrives for an appointment, you would need to ask for permission before revealing to the client what you are feeling. If the client shows any sense of discomfort, the agreed upon relationship should continue without overtly acknowledging the parallel world in which you are a child. If you can't manage to separate your "child" from the situation, and the client remains uncomfortable with the situation, offer the client the option of seeking another helper.

Sometimes the client may ask for help and yet, in another world, want friendship instead. Therefore, thinking you must simply help because that is what you think the person is requesting can be a mistake, and your helping hand can fail because the person may simply be lonely. Furthermore, in a nonlocal universe where the borders between you and the other are vague, you as a helper may not only be marginalizing the client's loneliness but your own as well. In this work, the other person's feelings are yours as well.

Any feelings of exhaustion and burnout you may experience as a helper are often due to marginalizing parallel worlds in which you are alone and quiet, or enjoying more of a personal life, or taking a vacation, or having time to dream. While vacation is important as a CR fact, it is also a parallel world occurring together with the world of everyday reality. To enjoy your work and not burn out on the one-dimensionality of Flatland, remember to invite in an awareness of other worlds, and bring those worlds into your work as much as possible. (For example, assume a more leisurely attitude while working.)

Multiple Role Awareness in Symptom Work

In previous chapters, we talked about how resolutions to the most difficult problems often lie in a parallel world, a hyperspace which has been marginalized. Because of the nonlocality of parallel worlds, your body will feel that marginalized parallel world. With lucidity, you become aware of this world and make changes there, indirectly influencing your client's symptoms (as well as your own).

By using your demon of lucid attention, you can bring hyperspaces to life for the benefit of all. To do this, use your awareness of multiple roles. Respect the agreed-upon relationship *and* simultaneously use your awareness to free yourself from the confining spaces of everyday reality to bring in fantasies of other worlds. Sense nonconsensual feelings and irrational flickerings and work with them, unbelievable as they might be.

For example, if a stern-looking friend or client tells you she has headaches, and you subtly feel pressured, then focus on the headaches and also focus on your feeling of being pressured. In that world where you feel pressured, you may discover an imagined critic who places pressure on everyone. The basic idea is that your pressure and that of the imagined critic create a polarity in nonconsensus reality that may be linked to the client's headaches. Because of the essentially nonlocal nature of nonconsensus reality, everything you experience is both in you and in the other.

In what follows, you will focus at first on resolving parallel world conflicts as if they were entirely within you (e.g., by playing out the struggle between the one being pressured and the critic). Then you will share the results and the process with the client. Finally we will see how the work relates to the presenting symptom.

Exercise: Nonlocal Therapy

This work can be done with anyone, any time, even while you are just chatting. Practice this exercise with a real or imaginary client. This work also can be done alone by imagining you are the client as well as yourself.

Imagine or do the following. When you are ready to interview your client, ask him or her to tell you about a body problem. (To simplify the gendered language, let's say this example involves a female client.) While talking, please use your awareness to notice what you are feeling in the moment.

Then explore your feeling experience, imagining it as a reaction to another role. To do this, imagine both roles. Notice what each role says to the other. Some people can do this best by staying in a relaxed, almost dreamy state of mind. In any case, use your lucid awareness about these roles, all the while staying open to the possibility that the client is a part of you. Again, while she is talking, notice her expressiveness and especially any and all of your own reactions to her. For example, Sally told me about her ongoing backaches. For some reason, as she spoke, I had the irrational feeling of being very "sunny," very optimistic, for no apparent reason. I thought, perhaps this sunny feeling is "just me." But then I realized that feeling must be in a parallel world and that I was reacting to something "in her." While she spoke, I noticed that she looked up at me in a very sad way, as if she were a sad child. I suspected the presence of a nonlocal field with two roles: One figure was a sunny parent, the other a hurt child.

Consider the other's expression and your reactions as roles, as a polarity in a parallel world. This polarity is one set of the multiple roles in your relationship that belong to both of you. However, in this training, play out the roles to begin with *as if they were only your own.* "Pick up" the field, take it on yourself. Use *your* fantasy and imagination and let your hands be puppets enacting these two roles interacting with one another. Let the roles speak to one another out loud. Then ask your (imagined) client for permission to reveal what you are experiencing.

While playing out the roles in front of your client, watch her feedback. If she seems fascinated or starts laughing, that is a hint you are on the right track. Keep enacting those roles until a resolution occurs. At this point, I imagined the sunny parent in my left hand and the sad child in my right. The child complained, "I am feeling so bad, and I hurt." Meanwhile the sunny parent (in the other hand) spoke lovingly to the child. "Don't worry, I am here." Before I—or rather, the sunny parent—could say more, Sally interrupted, saying, "How do you know that is my main problem? I never feel anyone loves me!" Without answering, I went on with my two hands talking to one another. The parent said to the child, "Whatever you do from now on, you will feel lots of love."

If the problem is not yet resolved in the parallel world of hands, puppets, and fantasies, go deeper. Get to the essence of the most difficult figure as quickly as possible. Find or guess the basic energy—the essence—of the troublesome figure, an energy that was present in a benign way before that figure became so dramatic. (To find the essence of a figure, *feel into* the figure and move your hand more slowly.)

I decided the most difficult figure was the hurting child. The child in my right hand spoke, "I am child! I cannot do so much in life, and I can't do things alone. I need love and support!" As the child spoke, I wondered what her essence was. I made the motions of the child less dramatically to feel the energy or essence. I felt the child in my hand, and as the child moved more and more slowly, I could sense the force of her dreaming. Its essence was spontaneity, being totally open to the universe and to the moment.

The "child" went on. "Appreciate me, I am really the very essence of life—spontaneity and play!" Before I could finish, my client burst out laughing, saying, "Yes, yes, the child's playfulness and spontaneity are the real me!"

After a few minutes, leave your fantasies in dreamland and now focus on the client's realities. Ask where the figures you "saw" are located in her physical body. Ask her to describe her experience, intuition, or imagination of the problem you have been portraying. I asked Sally where that hurting child and sunny parent were in her body. Immediately she said that the agonized child was her back. After some thought, she said the sunny figure was in her heart. She said that when I said the child is open and playful, her back felt better for some reason. "Something relaxed," she said.

Consider if and how the roles you just worked on are related to the client's experience of symptom creator and symptom receiver. This suggestion did not fit my client's experience. She needed to go no further. Her back relaxed; the cramp in her back muscles apparently dissipated. I had no chance to work further with her. This is a short story; she left my office without a backache.

If you have a CR identity of being a psychologically oriented helper, a next step might be to speak with an interested client about how to bring the discoveries to life. For example, how does the parallel world resolution want to be lived in everyday reality? A more medically oriented helper might ask, at this point, what

sort of allopathic, alternative, or complementary medical procedures might support the client's overall process the best.

The Universe As Your Body

At some point in the exercise, you may have felt that what you
were doing was not just about the client but also about yourself.
Nonlocality is the reason you do not know whether the work is
about you or the other. The work is about both and neither. Your
confusion is due to marginalizing the nature of nonlocality and
parallel worlds. Nonlocality leads to uncertainty about who is who
in dreamland. Definitive times and spaces belong only to the CR
"doctor" and "patient." In dreamland, roles are simply shared.

A creative and important aspect of nonlocality is the overlapping of personal boundaries in dreamland. This shamanic kind of
nonlocal experience is based upon the force of silence that
includes all the multiple dimensions, worlds, and roles in relationship. By sensing the problems "in the air" and trying to resolve
them there, you are focusing on the symptom's hyperspaces. The
problem in the client's body is not localized in there but is *everywhere*.[6] In a way, no one person has a problem; there is only ongoing awareness work, everywhere, anytime, all the time. Symptoms
belong to no one (except in CR).

Most of us, and especially scientifically oriented medical
helpers, sometimes need encouragement to open up to shut-down
feelings and understand them as sources of great information.
Every interaction around suffering creates and reveals parallel
world roles. If these are not taken seriously, they can become
obsessions, blotting out the CR relationship between doctor and
patient.[7]

In a nonlocal universe no one person is the "client" or the
"doctor." None of us really has feelings of his or her own; with
lucidity, you notice that we *share* feelings. Furthermore, if someone around you is stuck, then in some parallel world, you too are
stuck. Therefore, to help someone else, you need the very same
medicine. Each client brings you your own conflicts. Their

Rainbow Medicine is also what you need (just as your medicine may be helpful to them).

In an expanded and multidimensional view of reality, everything you notice is part of your body. In this view, we are seeds, or better yet inclinations and intentions, which unfold into stories in dreamland and in individuals like you and me in reality. We usually understand relationships as a CR friendship of some sort. However, from the viewpoint of other dimensions, our CR relationship is based upon our consent that you play one role, while I another, marginalizing the fact that in dreamland, we share the same story and all its roles.

Lama Anagarika's quote in the beginning of this chapter made the same point in this way: "To the enlightened man . . . whose consciousness embraces the universe, to him the universe becomes his 'body,' while the physical body becomes a manifestation of the Universal Mind."

Solving conflicts that appear in the moment to be your own or someone else's has nonlocal effects on everyone's body.

21 Nontoxic Lifestyles

. . . there is a universal flux that cannot be
defined explicitly but which can be known only
implicitly, as indicated by the explicitly definable forms and shapes, some stable and some
unstable, that can be abstracted from the universal flux. In this flow, mind and matter are
not separate substances. Rather, they are different aspects of one whole and unbroken
movement.

—*David Bohm*[1]

Your body is the battleground for opposing hyperspatial forces
seeking resolution. Care for your everyday CR body. Take the
medicines you need, find doctors who can help.

If your medicine is not enough, the battle proceeds overtly
and on a subatomic level requiring awareness of subtle, nonlocal
experiences. You may then need to understand your symptom
not as an enemy, but as an ally with an unpacked gift filled with

a rainbow of multiple experiences, dimensions, dreams, and mysteries.

Symptom As Enemy or Ally

This book suggests that there is no way around meeting the ally in those symptom experiences, a power you may have avoided until now. Explore flickering fantasies and feelings, notice subtle sensations, aches, pains, and pressures.

To begin with, work as if the symptom were local. Use your sensory-grounded awareness and study the body locations. Go deeply into the nature of the symptom, experience and imagine its creator. As a shaman, turn what seems to be a demon into an ally, or at least get to its essence; find the demon's secret, the force of silence that gave rise to the demon.

In the future, you can practice preventative medicine by remembering that flickering sensations of discomfort signal the need for more awareness and are the origin of possible body symptoms. The force of silence and the quantum mind initially appear as flickering sensations and later as dreamlike figures and a rainbow of parallel worlds.

From the viewpoint of consensus reality, symptoms are yours; they are in your body and connected to your history. But from another viewpoint, they come from nowhere. Just as particles can appear from the apparently empty space of a vacuum, symptoms can appear as if from infinity, from the force of silence. When you are reduced to near zero and your everyday mind is quiet, you can feel tendencies moving you along a given path—whether you call these tendencies collectively the Tao which cannot be said, or God, or the invisible pilot wave present at the beginning of the universe. If you choose to ignore this path, it appears in dramatic forms, sometimes in body problems or relationship difficulties.

The battle rages inside you, and the battle confuses your relationships. The battle is found in your family. Your community is the field of battle. The whole world is your body, your story.

Working at only one level makes the battle feel impossible and exaggerates its personal significance. The battleground is any and all levels of reality, and the battle is not only yours. In a nonlocal world, your symptoms are mine, and the medicine I need may be yours as well.

Why Me? Why Now?

While in the world of dreaming, we may understand that our experiences are nonlocal, but the everyday CR part of us may still wonder, "Why *me?*" "Why *now?*" "What did *I* do to deserve this battle?" Rainbow Medicine has an answer: Symptoms themselves contain the answer. Symptoms are coded messages from the vast landscape of universal interconnectedness that you experience as body problems.

The common denominator of all symptoms is awareness. Awareness is the ground of both subtle and excruciating signals. Body symptoms are not just pathology. They are Zen masters awakening your awareness of subtle, nano-like events.

Nontoxic Lifestyles

Marginalizing aspects of your life is toxic. Using awareness at each and every level creates a nontoxic lifestyle. You have more available energy, and you get to know parallel worlds. A nontoxic lifestyle is a lot of fun. Everywhere is your home, everything is filled with the unknown: your mind, your body, your relationships, your family, your community, and your world. Nontoxic lifestyles are comprised of awareness work that notices creativity in every moment, 24/7.

When something bothers you, use your awareness. Carefully notice the intensity of what you are doing. Then, with the same intensity, slow your movement down until you notice the seed, the force of silence behind your "doing." Then create Rainbow Medicine by letting that force move you.

PENO: Public Enemy Number One

Symptoms seem to win the battle when you believe they are only in your body. That's when your pain turns to agony, when medication and medical treatment seem insufficient. Symptoms threaten to kill you in the worst sense when you take the side of PENO, which is my acronym for Public Enemy Number One. PENO tells you that consensus reality is all there is. PENO says, "Forget the other worlds! You can't measure them. You can't prove they exist. Forget dreamland, forget your deepest tendencies, there is no quantum world; it's just math! There is no emptiness, no force of silence. There is only that which can be measured, medicated, seen on an x-ray, felt as a lump, measured with an instrument, and found in a virus!"

PENO says, "I am the way. The only things we can be certain of are centimeters in space, seconds of time, and grams of weight." PENO says symptoms are merely a matter of blood counts, diagnoses, x-rays, and genes. PENO is a downer denigrating that which cannot be formulated.

You cannot beat PENO, but you can use its energy. Get to the essence of PENO. Be precise with your awareness. Use your meticulously accurate, sensory-grounded awareness and focus on the consensus reality of the situation. With strict attention, don't just dream in the sense of being unconscious. Notice clearly what is happening. Then use your lucid awareness. Be a Maxwellian demon and let your lucidity penetrate the nature of irrational experiences and unspeakable feelings breaking open PENO's closed CR system and reversing the situation. Notice what is catching your attention. Act on it before PENO gets to it and labels it a "symptom."

Yes and No

Many parallel worlds will reveal themselves to you and can make you uncertain in CR. You want to know if you should fight or surrender, say yes or no, go this way or that, live or die. PENO tells you that you must choose one way. But from the viewpoint of the force of silence and dreamland, both yes and no, both right and wrong, are valid. Nontoxic lifestyles do not marginalize but accept that you are all worlds. You are simultaneously alive and dead. Good and bad are both correct. Don't fall for PENO's toxic lifestyle that has you identifying only with your CR self and standing against other sides of yourself.

You may agree or disagree with my conclusions. In a universe of parallel realities, all your arguments are bound to be correct in one of those realities—just as mine are correct in another.

Your Life Is None of Your Business

From the viewpoint of essence, your life is none of your business. You will eventually have to surrender CR to realize that the bottom line is that your life is up to the intentional field and the force of silence.

So take it easy and let it "do its thing." You get more done that way. Even small things are none of your business. From what you wear to what you believe in, events are up to that magnetic background that arranges flirts. Follow your deepest self. That creates the kind of backaction which might even rearrange your genetics, making you more coherent with your changing nature.

No child under the age of four has ever said, "I don't have time to follow my impulses—I'll wait till tomorrow." Children follow flirts right now, in the timeless here and now. PENO doesn't rule their lives, yet. With a beginner's Zen mind, you too can live in time and space as if they were filled with real tables and chairs, used in part by dragons and ghosts.

Someone asked me if all this means we should never make a plan. Nontoxic lifestyles include lots of plans; they are lived when they occur in whatever way is possible. When you think of tomorrow, don't kid yourself. That so-called tomorrow is happening right now, in this very instant.

PENO believes that time and life are its business; PENO is opposed to the style of letting things happen, of past and future being parallel worlds in the moment. Whenever PENO says, "There's not enough time now," you know it is right, but you are right as well. Time does not exist.

Rainbow Medicine in Organizations

Living and working with yourself and your loved ones will never be enough because of the effects of nonlocality. There is no place you can go to get away from this world. You can choose to not answer your mail, e-mail, or telephone. But you have nothing to say about the nano-like flirts you receive from infinity. You answer them before you know it.

Rainbow Medicine for organizations is simple. Support one side, then the other, then support all sides. Find the essence of the worst. In that "worst" role or person, deep in the essence level, is the thing that holds your group together—not the CR person, but his or her *essence* is what everyone needs; it's the bottom line of a community vision.

Do the same with your family members. Take all the conflicts onto yourself and find the essence of the most complicated figure. That is how to nourish yourself and others as well. Welcome polarities. Take one side; take all sides, and drop them for the essence. When the world and your community trouble you, remember nonlocal medicine and the idea that the community is a map of your body.

The Seeds of Possibilities

A dying Zen master, surrounded by weeping devoted students sadly lamenting his approaching death, suddenly hit them on the head with his stick and said, "Where do you think I am going when I die?"

My momentary answer to his question is that he is going nowhere and will be what he always was. Like you and me, with or without his CR body, he is the force of silence, manifesting as the essence of a story. We are the seeds of possibilities, the intent of a community.

Life and death, like space and time, are insufficient to describe our complete nature. In dreamland and the imaginary spaces of quantum physics and biology, we are both alive and dead. This means that we are dead when alive, and also alive when we are dead. That is one of the conclusions I must come to after studying the psychology, biophysics, and math of body symptoms.

The Quantum Source of Healing

At every moment throughout life, everything about our bodies is governed in great part by the same paradoxes ruling the quantum world. Perhaps the most wonderful of these paradoxes is that body symptoms contain their own amazing resolutions. Sensitive and lucid awareness reveals the transformative power of a quantum source of healing within even the most impossible symptoms.

There are many analogies and coincidences in how our bodies and minds connect to quantum physics. Just remember Bohm's pilot waves and the sense of guidance you felt working deeply on your symptoms. Parallel worlds mirror your various states of mind. The appendices include more of these analogies and connections. The links between psychology and physics offer the field of research a veritable treasure house, a whole universe of undiscovered insights. It seems inevitable that new kinds of biomedicine or rainbow medicines will emerge, integrating subjective experience and recreating what we call reality.

Until now, most of us have found or projected the cure for illness onto today's allopathic and alternative medical practices. Yet healing in the largest sense requires getting into sync with your deepest self. This synchronization process is partly a matter of your own awareness work. I have indicated in the foregoing chapters that getting in sync with yourself in-forms and reshapes your biochemistry, relationships, and group life. Using your awareness in symptom work can extend the sense of life beyond your wildest fantasies. The essence of symptoms frees you from time and space while planting you firmly on the ground. In this way, you may discover that symptoms are potential blessings.

APPENDICES

Introduction to the Appendices

My intention in the preceding chapters was to inspire the general reader to try new, practical approaches for working with symptoms. In these appendices, I wish to join those interested in exploring some of the fundamental ideas in science and psychology, conventional and alternative medicines, to go more deeply into quantum mind issues and the eventual unification of the sciences. May the following be a contribution to understanding some of the basic elements of this exploration.

These appendices are divided into three sections.

Appendix A: *Waves* focuses on the study of waves and wave theory. Here you will find information on the psychology and math of waves, and something about their applications in physics. A beginning theory of the quantum state crossover between psyche and matter is presented at the end of this section.

Appendix B: *Worlds* discusses Hugh Everett's many-worlds interpretation of quantum physics and his idea that observation splits reality in parallel domains.

Appendix C: *Minds* summarizes some of my ideas about the quantum mind.

Appendix A
Waves: The Quantum State Crossover

All matter is involved in a continual cosmic
dance. . . . All particles "sing their song,"
producing rhythmic patterns of energy.
—Fritjof Capra[1]

I love waves. I can't wait to get to the ocean and stare at how
the water rises and falls. When I see waves move in that endless
way, I can feel the pull of gravity between the moon and the Earth.
(The moon "tugs" on the Earth as it circles it, creating waves.)
Waves, waves, waves—everything moves up and down, day and
night. Considering the connections between waves, altered states
of consciousness, and quantum states is, for me, an exciting
endeavor.

Waves will help us connect what we call *body* and *mind* in
consensus reality. The quantum state crossover (chapter 9)

describes a potential connection between psyche and matter, what we used to call psychophysical or psychosomatic connections.

Pneuma, Strings, and Waves

Before going forward, let me go backward and ask you some elementary questions about yourself. What gives you the sense or idea that you are alive? How do you know that you are alive? Think about that question for a moment. Many people will say, at one time or another, that they know they are alive because they think and feel spontaneously, or because their bodies do different kinds of spontaneous things. Most people feel they are alive because they are breathing.

Let's say breathing is basic to your sense of life. Lack of breath is enough to make some fear they are going to die. Many meditation procedures connect you to your sense of breathing and the world of tendencies and origins of consciousness and life.

The periodic, rhythmic nature of breathing is usually further from your awareness than more (apparently) linear aspects of life, such as the passage of time or the sense of getting older. You probably identify yourself more with the linear passing of time then you do with the oscillations and periodicity of the changes of seasons, the movement from day to night, or the inhaling and exhaling rhythm of breathing.[2]

Nevertheless, we sense breath as life. For example, *pneuma*, sometimes translated as "spirit" or "life," was considered by early Europeans (especially those in the Gnostic tradition) as the vital substance, the essence of life. Too much or too little *pneuma* was thought to cause severe disorders.[3]

One of the crucial characteristics of the vital substance of life and breath is its wavelike nature. It is not surprising that our basic theories about matter and life and the universe are wave-like. As you know from chapter 19, in ancient China the first substance of the universe was called the Tao and was identified as a fundamental oscillation between opposite tendencies. Aboriginal Australians saw time as the period changes in the moon, and the transition between reality and the Dreamtime. In the last century, physics reconceived matter at the quantum level in terms of matter waves or quantum waves. More recently, the wavelike nature of matter has returned in the ideas of string theory.

String Theory

There are different theories of matter in physics. Quantum mechanics says that space can be broken up into quanta and parts. Relativity assumes space is continuous. To put these two theories together, physicists sought out solutions in hyper-spaces—higher dimensions—and developed string theory (and its extensions, "p-brane" and "M theory"). Physicists hope that hyperspatial thinking can incorporate both quantum mechanics principles and relativity theory via string theory.[4]

String theory proposes the existence of many dimensions; in fact, today's physics conceives of and uses between 10 and 26 dimensions. There are problems with the mathematics of string theory, and no one knows what these dimensions are made of, but the basic idea is that tiny vibrations, named strings, float through the universe. In principle, these pre-matter strings of vibrations are the basic stuff of the universe and give rise to the CR world.

It is helpful to think of a guitar string when thinking of these strings proposed by physicists. When the guitar string is stretched between two points, held under tension, and plucked, it creates tones, sounds, and waves. The universe's strings are not believed to be held down by anything, but they are imagined to be under tension and to hold energy. They even aggregate into the virtual waves of quantum mechanics. When strings become standing waves, our measuring equipment senses them as particles. String theories propose string *loops*, some of which open.

String theory says that the frequency of wiggles or vibrations enables open or closed loops to represent fundamental particles. Specific frequency patterns represent specific elementary parti-cles. Depending on the frequency of the vibrating pattern, the

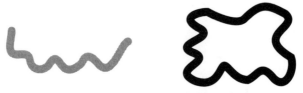

Figure A-1. String Theory: Open strings and closed loops.

string may appear to be what physicists have differentiated as quark, lepton, or electron particles.

Strings are considered to be more elemental than particles. The waves of the strings in string theory are more fundamental than what everyone has always thought was matter. What we thought were particles are now strings or waves. Point-like particles don't exist anymore. Now, string physicists say, "Let's relax our idea about particles being points; we can't measure them anyhow."[5]

The Psychology of Strings and Waves

Let's think about waves some more. Look at the two forms below, the point and the wiggly thing. What is the difference between the two forms for you?

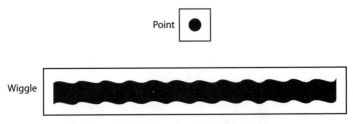

Figure A-2. The Difference between Points and Wiggles

Many people would say that the point is sharp and perhaps more static. The wiggle moves more (of course, points can move and standing waves can be static). I would suggest that the difference between points and waves is mirrored by the difference between *states* and *processes*. Much of our life activity is based upon points (or making points). Time and space are determined by points: *Be there at 5 P.M. Capetown is at a specific longitude and latitude.* We know that no one lives at that single point, but we nevertheless have a consensus about the existence of points. Let's say you are said to be 5'7". But if you have been sitting a lot, your back becomes compressed and you will measure a quarter of an inch less. Hang from a rope, and you will become taller. So what height are you?

You are a process, not a state. Furthermore, we make ap*point*ments which are usually points in time and place. *Time, location,* and *height* are nothing more than imagined particular points on a clock or measuring stick, but do they exist? Yes, they do exist as ideas in consensus reality. But in quantum physics, a point, like a particle, is more of a vision than a fact.

Most everyday CR communication is point-oriented. People are more likely to say, "Get my point," than they are to say, "Catch my drift" or "wave." When we speak of waves, we are usually referring to something more nonconsensual, such as, "We are on the same wavelength."

Fascinating Waves

Even the simplest wave—a regular succession of pulses—is periodic. Think about what happens when you pluck a guitar string. Its tone depends upon its frequency—that is, the number of times it vibrates per minute. Water waves, light, and sound are examples of periodic waves.

You can create a wave movement in a loose string by "waving" it, or by a pulse or series of tugs. A pulse or impulse can be large or small, even a tiny flicker. Your body is a pulsating medium. If you are very sensitive to your body, you can feel your own pulse or heart rate.

What is the origin of this pulse or life force? In chapter 7, I inferred that the quantum waves (and strings) are *just there* in the universe; they are the essence, the force of silence of the larger Being we are part of. As individuals, we can make pulses and new waves as we do in music; perhaps the whole universe makes little jitters or fluctuations in the zero-point energy field,[6] through which it pulses everything into life.

For the moment, let's stick to the pulses that occur in the math of physics. See the pictures below. A pulse is a general term for the motion creating any sort of general wave, whether it is real or imaginary.

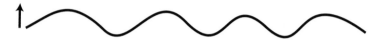

Figure A-3. Simple Periodic Wave

Below, we can see how a pulse is transmitted along a stretched flexible string tied to a wall. This is a simple kind of wave motion, as seen at time t_1, time t_2, etc.

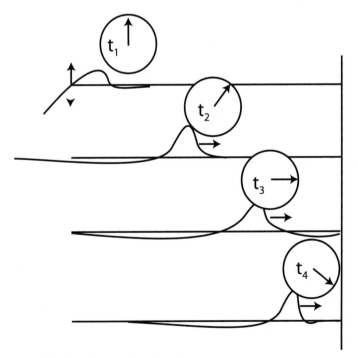

Figure A-4. Pulses Create Wave Motion

If pulses come from both ends of the string (let's say, because the pulse bounces, or is reflected, off the wall) instead of a pulse originating at only one end of the string, we notice something typical of all waves. Two waves coming from opposite directions add to or subtract from one another. They may add up to a bigger wave or cancel one another out. Scientists speak of this phenomenon in terms of how waves superpose themselves upon one another.

Superposition

Superposition, the way waves overlap, is a special property of waves that occurs whenever they meet. The way they add and subtract, the way they superpose, does *not* happen to particles, *only* waves. In consensus reality, particles bang and bump when they meet. But waves are different. They add (or subtract) and then go on their merry ways, more or less forgetting that they met one another head on. In my next diagram (figure A-5) of how two waves interact, one comes from the left and the other from the right.

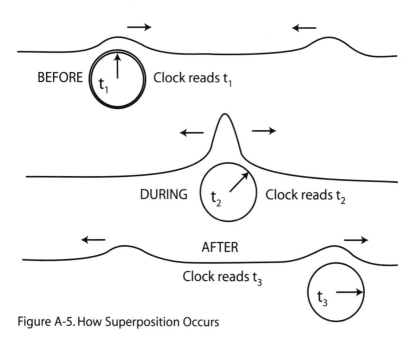

Figure A-5. How Superposition Occurs

Superposition occurs when they meet or intersect. Notice that after their meeting at t_2, the pulses at time t_3 are basically unchanged and continue to go on their way. Waves have an independent or separate nature. They interact, add, and subtract, but do not lose track of what they are.[7]

If the waves had had an opposite polarity instead of having the same size and shape, what would happen then? See the next diagram, where the waves actually cancel one another out as they pass through one another at t_2. Where did their energy go? The energy goes into the vibrations of the string.

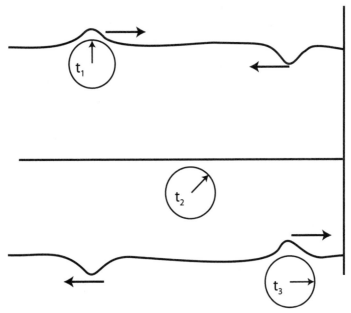

Figure A-6. Wave Cancellation

Waves relate to one another in a very different manner from particles. Waves add up (or subtract and cancel) when they meet, whereas particles bounce off one another. The path of particles after a meeting is altered. Waves continue on as before, as if they were relatively separate.[8]

Particles try not to let go during interactions; they are a bit like rigid people who bump and bang into one another when meeting. Waves are like more relaxed people who can add to or be subtracted from, but who afterward go on without having been substantially changed.

We humans are both wavelike and particle-like. If you criticize me, most of the time I behave like a particle and get indented and may bump back. If my awareness is focused on nonconsensus reality, I am more wavelike when criticized; I accept the situation—feel agreed with or corrected—and go on.

The same superposition happens inside us as outside in nonconsensus reality. For example, if one side of me says "yes" and the other says "no," then chances are I will just feel blank. (If I used awareness to notice what was happening, however, I would notice a dynamic inner balancing occurring at a point like t_2.)

My point is that inner experiences are wavelike processes; they superpose. Each wave or world tends to remain separate and relatively unchanged over time.

Superposition Principle

The superposition principle is a general rule.[9] Applied to wave phenomena such as water waves and quantum waves, this principle

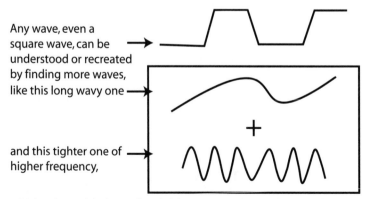

Any wave, even a square wave, can be understood or recreated by finding more waves, like this long wavy one →

and this tighter one of → higher frequency,

$+$

which, when added together (with many more waves), approximate the square wave above.

Figure A-7. A Superposition Example

says that the combined effect of any number of interacting waves at a point is the summation of the strengths (or amplitudes) of all the waves that are present at that given point. See the example of the square wave in figure A-7. which can be approximated by adding other waves together. The superposition principle says that when two or more waves move through the same region of space, the waves will superpose and produce a well-defined combined effect consisting of the sum of both waves. Waves maintain their integrity upon overlapping (i.e., without themselves being permanently changed).

I agree with Richard Feynman who said that the superposition principle (any wave can be understood as the sum of others) is the most amazing principle in all of math and physics. Since any wave (like the square one in the box) can be imagined to be a group of other waves, any particle with a wavelike representation can also be represented by a group of waves.

Physicists in the 1920s, such as Erwin Schrödinger who first discovered quantum waves (calling them "matter waves"), grabbed this principle and said, "Well, if any wave is the sum of many other waves, then any single wave—like a quantum wave for a particle—must have a lot of 'sub-waves,' each of which must represent separate quantum states of that wave/particle."

They were right! An object's main wave breaks down into sub-waves that represent its subatomic states. The overall wave function for an object is the sum of all of its sub-quantum states. In short, the subatomic states of an atom consist of the various ways in which it vibrates! In everyday language, we can say that the basic mathematical pattern of an atom—or any physical object for that matter—is the sum of all its possible quantum or dreamlike patterns.

Dream Fragments Are Sub-Waves

Schrödinger was a therapist in a way. Therapists like me think that a person only looks like a person in CR but is really a group of sub-personalities in NCR (nonconsensus reality). That is why therapists always suggest that knowing yourself means knowing your various parts and processes. Just look at your dreams. We know that even if you had a dream with five different fragments in it the night before—say, you dreamed about trees, dogs, your father, your sister, and a schoolteacher—that each of these figures or sub-personalities is needed to add up to the essential you. In your everyday reality, you don't see these dream substances; they are superposed, creating what we might call your overall glow or aura, your force of silence, the subtle pattern that drives you.

In dreamland, you have many sub-personalities, just like an atom has many quantum states. Each state, each personality, represents a tendency or possible real way in which you might behave under given circumstances.

Separable Worlds

Each wave is a separate or parallel world, a track you might take, which remains essentially independent of the other tracks you are on. You have likely experienced countless separable parts in your own life. You can be doing one thing while vaguely aware, at the same time, that you are dreaming or fantasizing or humming a tune about a different subject. Doing one thing while humming about another is an ordinary example of parallel worlds. The total you is a superposition of both worlds.

Waves and Particles

Now let's put some of these various views of matter together. Remember that in classical physics, and in today's medicine as well, a particle is still thought of as a particle, a chemical a chemical, and your body is a body. Now quantum physics and string theory have added the idea that particles and bodies are *clouds of probability* or simply waves.[10]

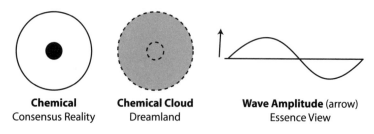

Chemical
Consensus Reality

Chemical Cloud
Dreamland

Wave Amplitude (arrow)
Essence View

Figure A-8. Evolving Pictures of Matter

We just learned that any wave is the sum of other waves. Recall that in the first chapters of this book, I discussed how David Bohm (and his predecessor, DeBroglie) saw the CR particle, such as an electron, as a sort of imaginary bit led about by its wave through space and time. Bohm imagined the quantum wave as a pilot wave.

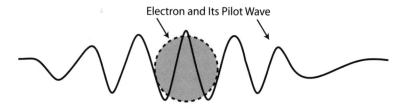

Electron and Its Pilot Wave

Figure A-9. Sketch of Bohm's Vision of Matter

Bohm's view of particles incorporates the virtual nature of matter which we experience in our bodies (the informational nature of the intentional field) and at the same time includes a picture of how we have consented to imagine matter and ourselves in consensus reality (e.g., as particles, objects, and people in time and space).[11]

Schrödinger suggested that the amplitude (or height) of a quantum wave contains the importance of that particular quantum state for the whole system.[12] When squared, this amplitude becomes a probability of things happening in everyday reality. This distance from trough to trough (wavelength) represents an individual frequency or tone of the virtual, immeasurable quantum states.

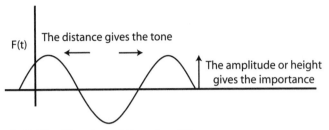

Figure A-10. The Meaning of Quantum Waves

Schrödinger's discovery of the wave equation is one of the great achievements of the twentieth century, encompassing much of physics and, theoretically, all of chemistry. It is a mathematical tool of great power for understanding the atomic structure of matter.

His first name for quantum waves was "matter waves," by which he imagined something material which could be eventually measured. These waves turn out to be immeasurable in the terms of consensus reality, but they are material in the sense of body-felt, body-sensed experiences. His intuitions about the subatomic realms are, in my opinion, intuitions about the dreambody's intelligence. Some call it the Great Spirit; others might refer to as the quantum mind. For Schrödinger, it was "matter waves."

The Quantum State Crossover

In this appendix I have suggested that the immeasurable quantum states of matter are analogous to and perhaps even the very same as the substates mentioned in our so-called psychology. At any moment, the quantum or pilot wave field, which I also refer to as the intentional wave field for experiential purposes, is moving us about, informing us in a manner similar to how Bohm imagined a particle is informed and transported by its pilot wave. This intent is the essence, the force of silence, manifesting as movement tendencies you feel in everyday life if you have developed your awareness, or when asleep, lucid and still.

As the force of silence emerges from the essence world into dreamland, it breaks into dream fragments. Just like quantum states (e.g., individual modes in which atoms vibrate), all fragments are essential contributors to our wholeness. In everyday reality, reflecting on dreamlike experiences gives us an approximate sense of our behavior, just as quantum states reflect and self-amplify, producing approximations of what will happen.

The simliarities between the ideas, patterns, and structures of psychology and subatomic physics create a connecting point where psychology, art, and sciences overlap. I call this section of overlap, where matter and psyche merge, the quantum state crossover.

Our usage of the old terms, matter and psyche, is diminishing, as is our usage of consensual terms such as time and space; they are too vague to serve the more exacting needs of research. As cultures change, these older terms will eventually fall away; after all, they are but forms emerging from the force of silence. If you focus on images, you get psychology; if you use your proprioception and meter stick, you get physics.

Only in CR can we speak of your proprioceptive feelings *interacting* with your real physical body. Interaction is a CR term that conceives of things in terms of separate points and connections. At the deepest levels, your feelings *are* your body. Separate worlds cross over. Quantum states and altered, dreamlike states of consciousness are two names for the same underlying reality. When this reality—call it the force of silence behind our nature, strings, or quantum waves informing matter—changes, it transforms the overall dreamlike patterns which guide us, though their effect upon specific local body symptoms is governed by uncertainty principles.

In any case, in a process-oriented science, something is correct when it is reasonable in consensus reality *and* in dreamland and refers to known facts, as well as to common human (possibly immeasurable) experiences. In Rainbow Medicine, we should be able to test *and feel* new ideas and theories. In the new scientific paradigm, an idea is correct if it can be tested in CR and experienced in consensus reality, dreamland, and in the world of tendencies.

This means that the reasonableness of concepts such as the force of silence, the correctness of the superposition of multiple substates, and the idea of the quantum state crossover can and should be eventually subjected to and refined by CR tests of the future.

Appendix B
Worlds: Everett's Many Worlds

There are various concepts physicists use to understand the mystery of the wave equation—why it needs to be amplified to produce probabilities and what happens to its parallel worlds once it has become real in everyday life.

Probably the best known construct is the Copenhagen interpretation of quantum mechanics. This interpretation implies that nonconsensual events, such as parallel worlds, are mathematical oddities and can be disregarded as imaginary and hence meaningless.

Psychologically, however, we know that we tend to highlight some experiences and call those real, even as we forget, ignore, or disregard others. We usually highlight the ordinary appearance of a friend and ignore slight changes in that friend which make no immediate sense to us. As observers, we have more power to create and hold onto realities (such as the everyday appearance of a friend), than we are usually conscious of.

Hugh Everett, while a Ph.D. candidate under John Wheeler in 1957, dreamed up an alternative to the Copenhagen understanding of how reality comes about through the power of the observer.[1] Everett was quite a dreamer, or so the gossip goes. Michael Price reports that "Everett, apparently, had a very intense manner, speaking acutely and anticipating questions after a few words. Oh, yes, a bit of trivia, he drove a Cadillac with horns."[2]

Everett viewed the observer in a more deeply democratic way than other physicists. According to Everett, quantum states are parallel worlds; all these worlds exist at the same time, though the one we are in is the most probable we will perceive and experience in CR. In other words, for Everett, parallel worlds are all real states. Thus at any given moment, in one world we can be alive, while dead in another.

Everett's concepts led me to the idea of marginalization. If we view all worlds as real, the world we agree on is simply the most probable world, the most likely one we shall observe. What happens to the others? Why don't we see them? My answer is that we marginalize the rest of the world(s), telling ourselves they don't exist, even though they are right there, beneath our focus.

Everett pointed out that when two systems are about to interact with one another, they enter into the same wavelength for the moment. One system then registers this wavelength as a measurement. At another moment, the observer can enter into another wavelength or another world with the observed. In this way, there is no collapse of the wave function (as in the Copenhagen interpretation); there are now as many worlds as there are quantum states of the entire system.

In psychology we know this concept well. One day we meet our friend, and we enter one world together. The next day, we interact in another world and are on a totally different vibration with that friend. In this way, we are all familiar with parallel worlds (as well as dual roles and multiple worlds in relationships). Just as music appreciation requires us to hear the various instruments and sounds in a symphony, the various tones and overtones of a song, so psychological and physics appreciation should now require us to tune in to the various worlds and their imaginary spaces and times.

Together with, or right next to each and every observation in the CR world, lie multiple universes. Around each of us lies a multitude of experiences and universes. Practice noticing them.

Appendix C
Minds: The Quantum Mind

Technical yet still popular aspects of the quantum mind can be found in Nick Herbert's *Elemental Mind*, Fred Alan Wolf's *Taking the Quantum Leap,* and Amit Goswami's *The Self-Aware Universe.* Also see my *Quantum Mind* for more on the psychological basis of physics, and Stuart Hammerhoff's research on the quantum mind in medicine.[1]

Here I summarize some of the many meanings I attribute to the term quantum mind.

The tendencies of the quantum realm, according to Werner Heisenberg, exist in a "strange kind of physical reality just in the middle between possibility and reality"—like feelings we experience as not being quite real but which surround everyday reality. Heisenberg said that "the atoms and the elementary particles themselves are not as real; they form a world of potentialities or possibilities rather than one of things or facts. . . . The probability wave . . . means a tendency for something. It is a quantitative version of the old concept of *potentia* in Aristotle's philosophy. It introduces something standing in the middle between the idea of an event and the actual event, a strange kind of physical reality just in the middle between possibility and reality."[2]

The quantum mind cannot be properly captured as a concrete picture. We know what people and stones and trees look like. However, we cannot easily imagine the quantum mind, because, like the math of quantum mechanics, this mind is not a thing that possesses one concrete image, like a chair. In fact, according to Niels Bohr, only reality is measurable. I call this statement the consensus reality assumption. The reality of the quantum mind is an NCR experience, a sense of an informing field or an intelligence guiding us in ways we can not always explain.

When something in us decides to observe the quantum mind, it takes on the characteristics of things in everyday reality. If we are careful in our observations, we notice that before "we" observe something, it flickers in our awareness, and we cannot be certain if the impulse to observe comes from it or from us. In other words, the quantum mind resides in the field between and beyond the ideas and objects that appear to us in CR.

The quantum mind is self-reflective and self-awakening. It seems to us as if nature is curious and self-reflective. The quantum mind is self-reflective; it repeats itself, creating the sense of solidity, reality, understanding, and wakefulness. In chapter 6 of his book *The Mathematical Foundations of Quantum Mechanics*, John von Neumann shows that awareness is a necessary (if hidden) assumption for quantum mechanics, buried within the concept of the observer. In his thinking, the fundamental ground of reality is math, not the objects it describes in CR. In other words, what we ordinarily think of as the real world is not the real one. That's why I call it consensus reality.

Events once connected are always connected. Schrödinger said that once two atoms have interacted, the possibilities and tendencies of one atom are mixed or entangled with another forever. This immediate, nonlocal interaction is very different from our everyday attempt to separate ourselves from others and from our feelings. Subtle NCR events are interconnected.

Space, locality, particle, and body are only CR forms of their

Quantum PHYSICS Zero-point energy	Process Oriented RAINBOW MEDICINE Essence	Analytical PSYCHOLOGY The Unconscious
Beginning of the universe	Force of silence	*Unus Mundus*
Quantum wave field	Intentional field	Psychoid unconscious
Self-reflecting waves	Reflecting flirts	
Nano-events	Flirts, pre-signals	
Math	**Dreamland**	**Dreams**
Subatomic states	Parallel worlds	Dream fragments
Superposition	Process	Meaning
Probabilities	Body feeling, fantasy	Archetypal images
Reality, Time, Space	**Consensus reality**	**Everyday life**
Observables	Signals, double signals	Behavior
Measurement	Awareness	Consciousness
Particles, objects	Body, mind, person	Ego, persona
	Process	Individuation

quantum-mind representations, which are everywhere. Nonlocal interconnectedness means that once a piece of your shoe rubbed off on a sidewalk in some town, you and that sidewalk are always connected. Bohm called the indivisible, connecting essence of the quantum world "undivided wholeness"—a characteristic supported by research into the so-called Bell-Aspect theorems and experiments.

Parallel worlds are simultaneously present. The quantum mind can be felt as the force of silence and appears in various separate worlds characterized by *coexistence.* That is, the parallel worlds of the quantum mind are *separate realities.* Each world remains essentially separate. They may temporarily overlap, but they apparently do not strongly influence one another.

The quantum mind has many spiritual and scientific names. Most scientists resist terms like the Great Spirit, or don Juan's Nagual, God, or the Tao; nevertheless, spiritual ideas, though largely rejected by our scientific training, form the NCR basis of science. I think of Einstein's famous statement, "I want to know God's thoughts . . . all the rest are details."

In analytical psychology, Jung would probably have identified the quantum mind with what the alchemists called the *Unus Mundus* (i.e., the One World). As did Wolfgang Pauli, Jung speculated that the unification between psychology and physics would happen through a *"tertium comparitionis"*—a third medium. I suggest that the preceding Rainbow Medicine terms are a contribution to the description of this third medium. The list in the table is not meant to be comprehensive. It is merely suggestive and meant to stimulate further thinking among physicists and transpersonal therapists of all kinds.

Where does the quantum mind come from and how did it begin? I have no idea. "How" and "where" are CR concepts and are less meaningful in the imaginary realms of dreamland. As far as the effects of nonconsensual awareness and consciousness on our body are concerned, measurement must contend with nonlocality. In principle, a change in awareness in one place creates change throughout the universe, both forwards and backwards in time. Thus, human beings and everything else contribute to co-creating the quantum mind.

It seems to me that under these circumstances, awareness of experiences, as well as mathematical beauty and measurements in time and space, will eventually become a governing paradigm interpreting the dreamland and the mathematic spaces of physics. CR measurements and mathematical rigor and proof have been useful paradigms until now. Nevertheless, it is time for a renewed and more inclusive consensus reality which includes multidimensional awareness. I predict that focusing and appreciating subjective body experience as a fundamental reality will have remarkable and positive effects upon health issues.

Endnotes

Chapter 1

1. In a speech in April 2001 at the Fermi National Laboratory, in which he scolds physicists for forgetting how to dream. Online at www.latimes.com/HOME/NEWS/METRO/t000056856.html.

2. See appendix C, "Minds: The Quantum Mind," for more on the connection of the quantum mind to physics and psychology.

3. In the appendices, I speak about how our sense of this field is the psychological analogy to the quantum potential of physics and its wave function. The force of silence is then the immeasurable pressure of this field, the guiding intelligence we subjectively experience moving us through life.

4. For psychologists, imaginary time would support the reality of myths and mythic concepts!

Chapter 2

1. *Frontier Perspectives* (The Center for Frontier Sciences at Temple University), Fall 2000, 9(2): 27.

2. In Pais, "Wolfgang Ernst Pauli," *The Genius of Science*. 2000.

3. This is my interpretation of quantum physics; see my *Quantum Mind* for more.

4. In his *Original Tao*, 1999, Harold D. Roth tells us that his discovery of material called "inward training" is derived from long-lost texts that preceded Lao Tze' s famous *Tao Te Ching*. In his review of ancient ideas, which are said to revolutionize our ideas about ancient Chinese philosophy and science, the Tao or "the Way's power" creates all things. This world is a concrete manifestation of the Way's power.

5. Ibid., p. 46.

6. See Sogyal Rinpoche, *The Tibetan Book of Living and Dying.*

7. Heisenberg (1958), *Physics and Philosophy,* chapter 2. "It should be emphasized, however, that the [wave or] probability function does not in itself represent a course of events in the course of time. It represents a tendency for events and our knowledge of events."

Chapter 3

1. This talk was given at the California Institute of Technology (Caltech) and first published in the February 1960 issue of Caltech's *Engineering and Science* (which owns the copyright) but has been made available on the web at www.zyvex.com/nanotech/feynman.html.

2. Robert Freitas describes the exciting work on integrating nanoscience with medicine in his *Nanomedicine.*

3. Ibid.

4. See my *Quantum Mind* for a discussion of his work. Also see Fred Alan Wolf's *The Quantum Leap,* and especially his *Parallel Universes* (pages 219-223) where he explains in detail Cramer's originally called reflecting "offer" and "echo" waves that pass between observer and observed, or between the observer and herself.

5. I describe the flirting tendency in greater detail in *Dreaming While Awake.*

6. David Bohm (1957), *Causality and Chance in Modern Physics.*

7. An Aboriginal man explaining the concept of a "dreaming place" to an anthropologist; original source unknown, quoted from *IONS Noetic Sciences Review,* September-November 2000, Sausalito, CA 94965.

8. See my *Quantum Mind* for a more complete discussion of conjugation.

9. In Indian philosophy *prana* refers to the body's energies. A central concept in early Hindu philosophy, particularly as expressed in the Upanishads, prana was the principle of vitality that survived as a person's "last breath" for eternity or until a future life. See Gopi Krishna, *The Biological Basis of Religion and Genius,* with an introduction by Carl F. von Weizsaecker.

10. Ibid. Weizsaecker connected the kundalini to the wave function's "probability amplitude" in quantum theory.

Chapter 4

1. See Michio Kaku, *Hyperspace: A Scientific Odyssey through Parallel Universes, Time Warps, and the Tenth Dimension,* 1994.

2. See Nima Arkani-Hamed, Savas Dimopoulos, and Gerogi Dvali's *Scientific American* article entitled "The Universe's Unseen Dimensions" for a vivid and entertaining description of higher-dimensional thinking connected to modern physics and technology. According the authors, "Our whole universe may sit on a membrane floating in a higher-dimensional space."

3. Thanks to Carl Mindell for pointing me to Jacques Lusseyran's work.

4. Jacques Lusseyran, *And There Was Light.*

5. Ellen Chen's translation, 1980.

Chapter 5

1. Richard Feynman, *The Character of Physical Law.*
2. See chapter 6 of my book *Shaman's Body* for more.

Chapter 6

1. Dalai Lama, *Freedom in Exile.*
2. In *And There Was Light: The Autobiography of Jacques Lusseyran.*
3. See my *Quantum Mind,* chapters 16–18.
4. See chapter 3 of this book, p. 28.
5. In their *Harvard Educational Review* article, "Cognition, Complexity, and Teacher Education," Davis and Sumara support relocating the seat of perception and perhaps life itself: "What if we were to reject the 'self'-evident axiom that cognition is located 'within' cognitive agents who are cast as isolated from one another and distinct from the world, and insist instead that all cognition exists in the 'interstices' of a complex ecology of organismic relationality?"
6. In his book, *The Tao of Physics.*
7. In *Starwave.*
8. This definition can be tested because it links life to reproduction and the tendency to recreate itself and others according to a specific chemical formula. For example, crystals divide and reproduce without nucleic acids, but in this definition a crystal would not be alive. It has no nucleic acids.

The concept of molecules and enzymes is a consensual one. In nonconsensual terms, a system that reproduces but has no visible nucleic acids is like a "ghost"—it is no longer alive in the physical sense but it does exist on other levels. In many places in the world, during special "days of the dead," it is believed that the dead come back to life and can be remembered. In fact, contact with the dead can ensure a healthy life for the person contacted. The idea that the dead are no longer alive is understandable. However, CR beliefs of the modern world marginalize subtle experiences and the belief systems of many peoples.

9. In chapter 5 of his *The Creative Cosmos: A Unified Science of Matter, Life and Mind,* The Club of Rome member Ervin Laszlo admirably pulls together many recent criticisms of Darwin's theory.
10. For example, people in coma have often been assumed to be unconscious or near death. However, with lucid attention to subtle signals, many people in comatose states have been known to come to life in very surprising ways, as I have reported in *Coma: Key to Awakening,* and as Amy Mindell reported in *Coma: A Healing Journey.*

Chapter 7

1. Bruce Chatwin, *The Songlines.*
2. Entelechy (from Greek *entelecheia*) is a sort of informing spirit that realizes or makes actual what is otherwise merely potential. Aristotle distinguished between matter and form, or the actual and the potential. He

thought that matter needed an essence to make it real. In living things, this essence appears as a "soul" or "vital function," called first entelechy of the living organism. (See the *Encyclopedia Britannica* for more on this topic.)

3. In his book, Paul Davies focuses on cosmology, gravitation, and quantum field theory, with particular emphasis on black holes and the origin of the universe.

4. See especially Bohm's *Atomic Physics and Human Knowledge,* pp. 58–59.

5. See the "Post Quantum Physics" of Jack Sarfatti on his web page www.qedcorp.com/pcr/pcr/.

6. The Taoist Dragon comes from Phillip Rawson Philip and Legeza Laszlo's *Tao: Eastern Philosophy of Time and Change,* figure 55.

7. Ibid. Figure 28, of Liu-hai, the Immortal.

Chapter 8

1. Michio Kaku, *Hyperspace: A Scientific Odyssey through Parallel Universes, Time Warps, and the Tenth Dimension.*

2. In appendix A, I discuss in greater detail the theory and experience of waves in psychology and physics, and how our psychology is connected to our biology.

3. See more about atoms in appendix A.

4. Those interested in dream work will notice how associating sounds and rhythms to figures is a "sentient" method of working with dreams.

5. This sum is the basis of Fourier's ideas. See appendix A for more on wave sums.

6. See my book *Dreambody.*

7. See appendix B, "Worlds: Everett's Many Worlds," to find out more about Hugh Everett. Also see Fred Alan Wolf's discussion of Everett's work in *Taking the Quantum Leap.*

8. Michio Kaku may have arrived at this thought as follows: Each quantum state or process is characterized by waves, which coexist simultaneously with one another, adding and subtracting as they pass, but not seriously disturbing one another's nature.

9. See my discussion of Hawking's ideas in greater depth in *Quantum Mind.*

Chapter 9

1. From the Sufi *Message of Hazrat Inayat Kahn: Music* (vol. 2, chap. 3). See also: www.sacramusica.org/elfrm.htm. Thanks to Amy Mindell for this reference.

2. See "Throat Singers of Tuva," by Theodore Levin and Michael Edgerton, *Scientific American,* September 1999. The Tuvas of Mongolia and Siberia are perhaps the best-known overtone singers today. Their pastoral music is connected to an ancient tradition of animism, the belief that natural objects and phenomena have souls or are inhabited by spirits. In the Tuvas' vitalist belief system, mountains and rivers manifest not only in the

form of their physical shape and location but also as the sounds they produce. The peoples of ancient India believed that the Earth itself was created from the sound "OM."

3. See www.nanou.com.au/songlines. There are ceremonial songs that pass on these stories. As the ancestors underwent various adventures, the laws for living and hunting skills were established. Their songs, stories, and paintings are intertwined. The land was literally "sung" into existence.

4. In his book, *The Galaxy on Earth*, Richard Leviton shows how to understand the Earth's subtle realities in terms of personal experience, grounding esoteric knowledge in mythology, history, and the observations of travelers.

5. I purchased this picture from her (#LI1) at www.nanou.com.au/song lines/.

6. The idea of this exercise was inspired in 2000 after meeting scientists from the U.S. government's Los Alamos National Laboratory in Sante Fe, New Mexico. They were very interested in how Amy and I had connected quantum physics to the body and expressed the view that this approach is about 15 or 20 years ahead of the times. They felt we were making interventions in the nanochemistry of the body. See Freitas's *Nanomedicine* for more on nanoscience in medicine.

7. I realized only after writing this book that a possible repercussion of the quantum state "crossover" would be a re-creation of what we call psychology and physics from a more unified viewpoint. My suggestion for this unified reformulation is to begin by viewing nature as having a quantum mind, that is, an awareness of minute, dreamlike motions and the capacity for self-reflection. This "mind" manifests at first as events in dreamland (composed of a mixture of real and imaginary events). In psychology, these events appear as the directions and tendencies of dreams, and in physics as the direction and tendencies of matter and light in the space of complex numbers. In a future book, I will explain the details of how vectors in dreamland can be seen to reflect virtual particle paths in terms of Feynman elementary particle diagrams. In any case, according to this theory, these psychophysical dreamland vectors self-reflect producing consensus reality thereby making quantum physics and dream psychology "parallel worlds."

Chapter 10

1. See Nadeau and Kafatos, *The Non-Local Universe: The New Physics and Matters of the Mind*, p. 36.

2. Pierre Morin, M.D., from Portland, Oregon, in his interesting doctoral dissertation (2002) for the Union Institute in Cincinnati, Ohio, *Rank and Salutogenesis*, assembles statistics indicating that a community's belief system (as shown by its judgment of rank) influences the health of individuals.

3. See my *Quantum Mind*, p. 194.

4. According to Sheldrake in his *The Presence of the Past*, "Morphogenetic fields differ radically from electromagnetic fields in that the latter depend on the actual state of the system—on the distribution and movement of charged particles—whereas morphogenetic fields correspond

to the *potential* state of a developing system and are already present before it takes up its final form." He goes on to say, "Chemical and biological forms are repeated not because they are determined by changeless laws or eternal Forms, but because of a *causal influence from previous similar forms.* This influence would require an action across space *and time* unlike any known type of physical action." He says, "Past fields influence present ones by a non-energetic transfer of Information." Therefore, while physically real, they are not like the fields physics knows, involving instead "a kind of action at a distance in both space and time"—action which does not decrease over distance in space or length of time.

5. See discussion of nonlocality in my *Quantum Mind* and appendix C of this book.

6. *The Non-Local Universe: The New Physics and Matters of the Mind.*

7. The experiment resulting in quantum entanglement, or interconnect-edness, is sometimes called the "unity of the world" or the Bell experiment. This experiment showed that the photons from a given source of light are interconnected. Like all other quantum phenomena, light sometimes acts as particles and sometimes as waves. Imagine, for example, a neon lamp giving off light. A pair of light photons emerges from the neon lamp, with the photons radiating away from one another. One photon goes in one direction and the other goes in the opposite direction. An amazing experiment showed that whatever happened to one particle seemed to be connected to what happened to the other particle, regardless of how far apart they were or how long they had been separated. Bell's theorem (which John Stewart Bell wrote in 1964, "On the Einstein Podolsky Rosen Paradox in *Physics* 1: 95–200) proved that the chances for spin correlation for local hidden variables were constrained and exceeded by the quantum theoretical spin correlation function. This implies that quantum phenomena are inherently nonlocal, although it leaves open the possibility of nonlocal hidden variable theories as alternatives to quantum theory. Since the experimental verification by Allan Aspect in 1982, physicists are in general agreement about nonlocality.

8. See my *Sitting in the Fire.* This work is a development of a commonly used psychodrama technique developed by Jacob Moreno in the 1920s. In this method, individuals act out the dreamlike atmosphere of other individuals or small groups.

9. See my *The Deep Democracy of Open Forums: Practical Steps to Conflict Prevention and Resolution for the Family, Workplace, and World* for examples of how group process influences cities.

10. I tell different "real" stories about such moments in my book *The Deep Democracy of Open Forums: Practical Steps to Conflict Prevention and Resolution for the Family, Workplace, and World.*

11. See chapter 1 of my *Dreaming While Awake.*

Chapter 11

1. See Larry Dossey, *Healing Words.*

2. From Kircher's *Oedipus Aegyptiacus.* The ornamental border con-

tains names of animal, mineral, and vegetable substances. Their relationship to corresponding parts of the human body is shown by the dotted lines. This art is reprinted with permission from the Philosophical Research Society, copyright 1996.

3. See Richard Wilhelm's translation of the *I Ching, Book of Changes*.

4. Here I must mention a paper by a colleague, Dr. John Johnson, "Environmental Justice for All: Principles and Practices for Conflict Resolvers," in *AcreSolution*, Summer 2002. The article pinpoints how environmental issues are inherently relationship matters of social and psychological rank.

Chapter 12

1. See Stephen Hawking's website: www.hawking.org.uk.

2. See pages 91–100 of my *Quantum Mind* for more on imaginary numbers.

3. See www.hawking.org.uk/lectures/bot.html.

4. Ibid.

5. See Derek A. Long, *The Raman Effect*, p. 385.

6. Cramer discusses the Einstein-Podolsky-Rosen experiments with nonlocality (i.e., enforcement of correlations between separated parts of an entangled quantum system, across space-like separations) in his "Quantum Nonlocality and the Possibility of Supraliminal Effects" (Proceedings of the NASA Breakthrough Propulsion Physics Workshop), August 12, 1997.

7. According to Cramer, "It (the reflection process) is a two-way contract between the future and the past for the purpose of transferring energy, momentum, etc., while observing all the conservation laws and quantization conditions imposed at the emitter/observer terminating 'boundaries' of the transaction." Quantum theory is nonlocal because "the future is, in a limited way, affecting the past" (at the NCR level of correlations between quantum waves).

Chapter 13

1. See Rupert Sheldrake, "Part I. Mind, Memory, and Archtype: Morphic Resonance and the Collective Unconscious," and www.sheldrake.org/articles/pdf/44.pdf.

2. A highly alternative, informative, and stimulating critique of genetics and genetic engineering has been written by the courageous Mae-Wan Ho, *Genetic Engineering: Dream or Nightmare?* Continuum Publishing, New York, 1998.

3. Ernie Rossi in his 2002 book on the psychobiology of gene expression *The Psychobiology of Gene Expression: Neuroscience and Neurogenesis in Hypnosis and the Healing Arts* says that there is no longer a "may" about it—there is a feedback connection apparent at the molecular level. He discusses "gene expression . . . a new concept in psychobiology bridging brain growth, behavior, and creative human experience." (p. 3.) Rossi also proposes that "the wave equation . . . is a source of the psychobiology of gene

expression, neurogenesis, and healing." (p. 29.) He presents research about two new classes of genes: "immediate early genes" and other types that respond throughout the circadian cycle to environmental fluctuations. The *activity* group, for example, responds to exercise by initiating a cascade of neurogenesis-related processes.

4. Rossi, op. cit., discusses cutting-edge work in neurogenetic research and combines it with the practice of optimizing gene expression and neurogenesis to facilitate brain growth and healing via creative experiences in the arts and sciences and therapeutic hypnosis. See also Mae-Wan Ho's 1998 *Genetic Engineering: Dream or Nightmare?* for an excellent update on connecting physics with genetics.

5. Physical methods are constantly being developed to produce and repair genetic accidents. Perhaps even nanorobots will offer help to us in the future.

6. This dream friend had a meaningful personal message for the dreamer I cannot repeat here.

Chapter 14

1. Thich Nhat Hanh, *The Heart of the Buddha's Teaching*.
2. David Bohm, *The Undivided Universe*.
3. This analogy remains to be affirmed independently by other researchers. There are many questions waiting to be answered. How much can we predict about our bodies from our dreams, and what is the exact relationship between such predictions and probabilities gained from genetic information? What do dreams tell us that genetics does not, and what does genetics imply that we cannot find in dreams?
4. For more information, see Jung's *Psychology and Religion* and his *Psychology and Alchemy* (vols. 11 and 12 of his *Collected Works*).
5. As far as I can remember, Miss Una Thomas recorded "Kinderträume" from a seminar on dreams given by Jung at the E.T.H. in the 1920s in Zurich. Una was 90 when I met her in Zurich in the 1960s. She was definitely one of his most creative students!

Chapter 15

1. *Tao Te Ching*.
2. See Thich Nhat Hanh's overview of Buddhism in his 1998 *The Heart of the Buddha's Teaching*.
3. The Eightfold Path includes: 1) right understanding—faith in the Buddhist view of existence; 2) right thought—trying to practice Buddhism; 3) right speech—avoidance of falsehoods, slander, or abusive speech; 4) right action—abstention from killing, stealing, and hurtful sexual behavior; 5) right livelihood—rejection of certain kinds of work which do not conform with Buddhist principles; 6) right effort—development of good mental states and avoidance of bad ones; 7) right mindfulness—awareness of the body, feelings, and thought; and 8) right concentration—meditation.

Chapter 16

1. Richard Feynman, *The Character of Physical Law*.

2. To resolve strong cravings, spiritual traditions suggest giving yourself over to some higher power. Alcoholics Anonymous, AA, was founded upon C. G. Jung's idea that addictions and cravings are indicators of the deeper need for a relationship to "a higher power."

3. I explain these virtual particles in some detail in chapters 33 and 34 of my *Quantum Mind*, which is why I mention only a few of the more interesting details here.

4. Feynman's amazing concept of "virtual particles" blends relativity theory, principles from quantum mechanics, and electric field theory. Although not perfect, it is still the best theory in many ways. Newer hypotheses, such as superstring theory, may eventually supercede QED, but these new theories have a long way to go before they can tell us as much about the world as QED.

5. That is, because the two electrons "exchange" photons somewhat like two ice skaters on a pond might "exchange" or throw a ball to one another. (The ball represents the virtual photon that transfers momentum between the skaters, resulting in the skaters' repulsion from one another.)

6. According to the Heisenberg uncertainty principle, a particle's lifespan is determined by the expression $Et > h$, with E energy, t time, and h Planck's constant. So a particle with any energy can pop into existence for a short amount of time, as long as it does not violate the above relation. The higher the energy, the shorter-lived the particle.

Chapter 17

1. Since telomerase creates longer life in the cells, you might think that in the case of cancer, wherein cells go on and on in their growth, there might be *too much* telomerase. That thought turns out to be correct: Something switches on that enzyme, which seems to be overproduced in the case of cancer.

2. See, in particular, Carlos Castaneda's *Journey to Ixtlan*.

3. I am thankful for the permission of www.buddhanet.net for the use of these wonderful pictures. The Ten Ox-Herding Pictures apparently stem from the Ch'an master in the Sung dynasty of China (1126–1279 C.E.) and have spiritual roots in the early Buddhist texts. A graphic designer, Hor Tuck Loon, has given these pictures a contemporary treatment. See www.buddha net.net/oxherd1.htm.

Chapter 18

1. Roger Penrose, *Shadows of the Mind*.

2. Entropy is a measure of the unavailability of energy to do work in a system.

3. Thermodynamics is the study of the rules that govern how energy transforms from one form to another, how heat moves, and how usable energy becomes more or less available. "Available physical energy" can be directly converted into work. This energy is also referred to as usable or "ordered"

energy, in contrast to unusable or "disordered" energy (such as heat) that cannot be directly converted into work.

4. *Deteriorate* means that all usable forms of energy will be converted into unusable forms, such as heat (hence the reference to the "heat-death of the universe"). There is ongoing debate about whether or not the universe is truly closed. According to recognized leaders in the field, L. D. Landau and E. M. Lifshitz, the universe is not exactly a closed system if gravity is considered a dynamic "external" condition. Using their argument, our awareness could be an external, or at least nonlocal, condition as well.

5. For example, if your city were a closed system, then each building and its environment of heat, light, and matter moving through it would be a subsystem plus its environments.

6. Maxwell imagined two volumes of gas in a container, separated by a partition and having the same temperature at the outset. By noticing the faster molecules and opening the door in the partition between the volumes to allow them to go to one side, one volume could get warmer because of the raised speed of the molecules. In this way the demon could create order out of the disorder that is characteristic of gasses in equilibrium, at the same temperature.

7. It seems likely to me that spontaneous cases of healing involve lucid awareness that resolves inner conflict.

Chapter 19

1. See Lynn Caporale, *Darwin in the Genome*, p. 101.

2. These words from the Persian Baha'i mystic first appeared in *Some Answered Questions* in 1908, published by Kegan Paul, Trench, Trubner & Co. Ltd. The first U.S. edition was published in 1918.

3. I am thinking, in particular, of the quantum paradox referred to as "Schrödinger's Cat," in which the cat can be both dead and alive in the quantum world before observation. The basic idea is that the separate states of life and death are present as parallel worlds, even though the observed CR state of life (or death) excludes those worlds.

4. "Bardo" is a Tibetan term meaning "phase," referring to phases in everyday life, in the time near death ("light," "hungry ghosts," etc.), as well as after physical death has occurred. See Sogyal Rinpoche's *The Tibetan Book of Living and Dying* for more.

5. See my *Coma, Key to Awakening*.

6. Camille and Kabir Helminski, translators of *Rumi: Daylight*.

7. Aging-related loss of memory in many people is loss of what you intended to do. You forgot "why" you were doing something. A process oriented view of such memory loss is that you "need" to let go of knowing why you intended to do something and let "it" move you, let the subtle "tendencies" and force of silence create life.

8. See my *Coma, Key to Awakening*, pp. 33 and 34.

9. David Nankervis's interview with Lewis O'Brien, "We're Built Like a Giant Kangaroo," *Adelaide Times*, November 1996.

10. See my *Coma, Key to Awakening* for more such case material.

11. See Reggie Ray's wonderfully lucid *Indestructible Truth*.

12. See Amy Mindell's *Coma, A Healing Journey* for descriptions of "hands-on" work with the dying.

13. I discuss Aboriginal mythology in the first chapter of my *Dreaming While Awake*.

14. See Frank Fiedeler's work www.lunarlogic.de/Frank/introduction.htm.

15. See Wilhelm's (1981) *I Ching*, p. 265.

16. See *Causality and Chance in Modern Physics*, p. 11.

Chapter 20

1. See *The Quantum Self*, p. 132.

2. In his seminal book *The Tao of Physics*, Fritjof Capra quotes Lama Anagarika, of the Govinda Foundations of Tibetan Mysticism. See Capra's book, p. 305.

3. This demon is a description of a missing feature in quantum physics needed to explain why self-reflection appears in quantum wave theory. Without the universe's self-reflection ability, there might be no universe. Amit Goswami has rewritten an enlightening book, *The Self-Aware Universe,* on this topic. He uses the word *consciousness,* where I use *lucidity.*

4. I discuss signal exchanges in my *Dreambody in Relationships.*

5. In a medical or therapeutic setting, the most probable role pair is that of doctor-therapist and patient-client. The particular roles and worlds we enter together depend upon who we are, what we are doing, and the nature of the moment. Thus, a "dual relationship" for a clinical helper is any relationship which is not clinical. For example, a dual or multiple relationship would mean that in addition to being someone's therapist, you are also a supervisor, teacher, or friend.

Dual roles are the source of much discussion in the therapeutic communities today. Generally speaking, any role beyond the clinical is regarded as a problem in a therapy setting if it influences the therapist's objectivity. Rainbow awareness supports mainstream views. However, with or without rules, "objectivity" can *never* be completely achieved because the observer is *always* "entangled" with the observed in non-consensual reality (e.g., at the quantum level and in dreamwork). Therefore parallel-world awareness work in relationship will always be essential.

6. For example, in my *The Shaman's Body*, I tell how one Kenyan shaman couple explained their work. The couple visit once with their "clients" and then send them home. Then the couple go into a trance and solve the client's problems there. The antiquity and belief in shamanism indicate that it "works" more frequently than the modern CR observer might believe at first.

7. Multiple role "rules" are important because they validate and try to protect the helper-client relationship. However, rules need enforcing in the first place because of lack of awareness around the use of power in connection with roles.

Chapter 21

1. *Causality and Chance in Modern Physics,* p. 11.

Appendix A

1. Fritjof Capra, *The Tao of Physics,* pp. 241–242.

2. Though we experience our watches as moving forward in time, the experience of time may contract or expand for observers of time who are in frames of reference that are moving relative to one another. Furthermore, Einstein's space-time curves unequivocally demonstrate that we should never expect time to be linear.

3. See *Encyclopedia Britannica* on "Dualism" and the subtopic, "Life and Death."

4. For a simple overview of string theory, see Dr. Patricia Schwarz's "Official Superstring" website, www.superstringtheory.com/basics/index.html.

5. In his *Universe in a Nutshell* (pp. 54–59), Stephen Hawking speaks of updated theories that integrate quantum mechanics with relativity theory. In this book, he speaks in accessible language of the generalizations of string theory, "p-brane theory," and "M theory," which encompass all of the strings and their multidimensional counterparts, p-branes. As a "positivist," he says that since math is useful, we should use it and think about it without getting caught in the debate about its being "real" or not. This pragmatic viewpoint allows him to think of imaginary time and imaginary time concepts.

My viewpoint is that all theories are psychological; they come from our essence and unfold in terms of our dreams, the math we conceive, our hopes and visions, the stuff of everyday reality. So the hypothesized vibratory nature of quantum mechanics and its updated version in terms of string theory stem from the wavelike character experienced in our psychology—which we feel as body experiences such as kundalini and tendencies or nano-movements.

6. Zero-point energy is the energy remaining (in a substance) at absolute zero, -273°C, the temperature at which matter stops vibrating. This energy still exists because, according to quantum theory, a particle oscillating with simple harmonic motion does not have a stationary state of zero kinetic energy. The uncertainty principle does not allow such a particle to be at rest at exactly the center point of its oscillations. Hence, there is always energy (a zero-point) even when things seem totally empty.

7. At least, not in the simplest situations illustrated here.

8. When two or more waves are superimposed, scientists speak of the "net wave displacement," which is the sum of the displacements of the individual waves. Since these displacements can be positive or negative, their sum (or net displacement) can either be greater or less than the individual wave displacements. The former case is called constructive interference, and the latter is called destructive interference. Water waves, light waves, and quantum waves all interfere with one another. Interference is a consequence of the superposition principle.

9. For so-called linear systems. For example, water is more "linear" than a very viscous material. Waves dissipate unless they propagate though a "perfect" (or frictionless) medium.

10. In physics, the connection between waves and particles is established through the calculation of the probability of finding a particle in a given spot and time. This calculation is arrived at by squaring the normalized

amplitude of the wave function of that state. To do this, you take the height (or amplitude) of a wave and multiply it by itself to arrive at the probability that there is a measurable "particle" in consensus reality.

11. In his excellent book *Einstein's Moon* (pages 148 and following), David Peat discusses Bohm's thinking in an elemental non-mathematical manner. Though Bohm's basic math is consistent with mainstream interpretations of physics, Peat points out how some physicists, without completely understanding Bohm's ideas, did not accept his interpretation of quantum mechanics, because in Bohm's view, the picture of a particle remains more or less "a particle." Its wave function, which Bohm calls "the quantum potential," becomes a new kind of "in-form-ation" or nonlocal guiding force. Though the quantum potential is a causal and exact equation, the path of the particle is indeterminate because the slight changes in the values of the surroundings create slight changes in the quantum potential. Bohm later expanded his "causal" interpretation, retaining the essential indeterminacy of the particle's path (due to the sensitivity of the quantum potential).

Arguments over the philosophy of physics and the interpretation of wave functions are not as important to me as their connections with the psychology of awareness and psychological experience. Nonlocal, immeasurable fields can be "felt" as intimate and close, though in CR they may connect very distant objects. Unlike the fields of physics, such as a magnetic field around a magnet, the essence feeling or the quantum potential's informative quality does not decrease as things get more distant. A magnetic field, on the other hand, loses its power over a piece of iron as the magnet and piece of iron separate from one another. The quantum potential or guiding wave exerts a subtle informative "force" which may be "in back of" other real fields, such as magnetism and gravity, which can be measured. That is why I have called the quantum potential and its wave function "the force of silence," the apparently immeasurable subtle pressure or intelligence which we subjectively experience moving us.

12. A quantum state is a state of a quantized system described by its quantum numbers. For example, hydrogen has four such quantum numbers, 1,0,0, and 1/2, describing characteristics of the electron (its specific energies and spins).

Appendix B

1. See www.hedweb.com/everett/everett.htm for Michael Price's "The Everett FAQs"—great insights into Everett.

2. Ibid.

Appendix C

1. His website, listserv.arizona.edu/archives/quantum-mind/ is a good place to get updated on the applications of quantum mind theories to bio-computers and medicine.

2. See a good overview of Heisenberg's work in Nick Herbert's excellent *Elemental Mind*, pp. 146–178.

Bibliography

Abbott, E. 1952. *Flatland*. New York: Dover. (The original publication was in 1884 [Seeling and Co.], and the most recent Dover Thrift Edition appeared in 1992.)

Abdu'l-Baha. 1908. *Some Answered Questions*. (Republished by Kegan Paul, Trench, Trubner & Co. Ltd. London. The first U.S. edition was published in 1918.)

Arkani-Hamed, Nima, Savas Dimopoulos, and Gerogi Dvali. August 2000. "The Universe's Unseen Dimensions." *Scientific American*. Vol. 282, Issue 8, p. 62.

Arye, Lane. 2002. *Unintentional Music: Releasing Your Deepest Creativity*. Charlottesville, Va.: Hampton Roads. www.hrpub.com.

Batchelor, Martine, and Stephen Batchelor. 1995. *Thorson's Principles of Zen: The Only Practical Introduction You'll Ever Need.* Audio cassette, #0-7225-9926-9, Thorsons Audio/National Book Network. www.nbnbooks.com.

————.1996. *Walking on Lotus Flowers: Buddhist Women Living, Loving, and Meditating*. London and San Francisco: Thorsons, HarperCollins.

Beller, Mara. 1998. "The Sokal Hoax: At Whom Are We Laughing?" *Physics Today*. January 1997, p. 61, and March 1997, page 73.

Bohm, David. 1984. *Causality and Chance in Modern Physics*. London: Routledge and Kegan Paul. (First published in 1957.)

Bohm, David, and Basil Hiley. 1993. *The Undivided Universe: An Ontological Interpretation of Quantum Theory*. London and New York: Routledge.

Bohr, Niels. 1958. *Atomic Physics and Human Knowledge*. New York: John Wiley.

Caporale, Lynn. 2002. *Darwin in the Genome: Molecular Strategies in Biological Evolution*. New York: McGraw-Hill/Contemporary Books.

Capra, Fritjof. 1999. *The Tao of Physics: An Exploration of the Parallels Between Modern Physics and Eastern Mysticism*. 4th Ed., updated. Boston: Shambhala.

Castaneda, Carlos. 1972. *Journey to Ixtlan*. New York: Simon and Schuster.

Chatwin, Bruce. 1988. *The Songlines*. New York, Harmondsworth, England: Penguin Books.

Chen, Ellen. 1989. *The Tao Te Ching: A New Translation and Commentary*. New York: Paragon House.

Chopra, Deepak. 1998. *Ageless Body, Timeless Mind*. New York: Random House.

Cramer, John. 1997. "Quantum Nonlocality and the Possibility of Supraliminal Effects." Proceedings of the NASA Breakthrough Propulsion Physics Workshop, Cleveland. Cleveland, Ohio, August 12–14, 1997.

Dalai Lama. 1990. *Freedom in Exile*. New York: Harper Collins.

Damasio, Antonio R. 1999. *The Feeling of What Happens: Body and Emotion in the Making of Consciousness*. New York: Harcourt Brace.

————. 1999. "How the Brain Creates the Mind." *Scientific American*, 281, 6 (1999): 112–117.

Davies, Paul. 1999. *The Fifth Miracle*. New York: Simon and Schuster.

Dossey, Larry. 1993. *Healing Words*. New York: Harper Collins.

Encyclopedia Britannica 2001. (See especially its CD ROM version, available from www.britannica.com.)

Feynman, Richard P. 1966. "Notes on the Beginning of Nanoscience." Caltech's Engineering and Science website, www.zyvex.com/nanotech/feynman.html.

————. 1967. *The Character of Physical Law*. Cambridge, Mass.: MIT Press.

Freitas, Robert A. 1999. *Nanomedicine. Vol. I: Basic Capabilities*. Austin, Texas: Landes.

Godwin, Joscelyn. 1979. *Athanasius Kircher: A Renaissance Man and the Quest for Lost Knowledge*. London: Thames & Hudson.

Goswami, Amit, with R. E. Reed and M. Goswami. 1993. *The Self-Aware Universe: How Consciousness Creates the Material World*. New York: Tarcher/Putnam.

Gould, James L., and Carol Grant Gould. 1988. *Life at the Edge*. New York: Freeman and Co.

Govinda, Lama Anagarika. 1973. *The Foundations of Tibetan Mysticism*. New York: Samuel Weiser.

Grimm's Fairy Tales. London: Routledge and Kegan Paul, 1980.

Hammeroff, S. R. 1994. "Quantum Coherence in Microtubules, a Neural Basis for Emergent Consciousness?" *Journal of Consciousness Studies*, 1: 91.

————, and Roger Penrose. 1996. "Orchestrated Reduction of Quantum Coherence in Brain Microtubules: A Model for Consciousness." In S. Hameroff, A. Kaszniak, and A. Scott (eds.), *Toward a Science of Consciousness: The First Tucson Discussions and Debates* (p.115). Cambridge, Mass.: MIT Press.

Hanh, Thich Nhat, 1998. *The Heart of the Buddha's Teaching: Transforming Suffering into Peace, Joy, and Liberation; the Four Noble Truths; the Noble Eight Fold Path, and other Basic Buddhist Teachings*. Berkeley, Calif.: Parallax Press.

Hawking, Stephen. 1993. *Black Holes and Baby Universes, and Other Essays*. New York: Bantam Books.

———. 1999. Public lectures at www.hawking.org.uk/text/public/public.html.

———. 2001. *The Universe in a Nutshell*. New York: Bantam Books.

Heisenberg, Werner. 1958. *The Physicist's Conception of Nature*. New York: Hutchinson.

———. 1959. *Physics and Philosophy*. George Allen and Unwin Edition.

Helminski, Camille, and Kabir Edmund Helminski. 1990. *Rumi: Daylight: A Daybook of Spiritual Guidance*. Putney, Vt.: Threshold Books.

Herbert, Nick. 1993. *Elemental Mind: Human Consciousness and the New Physics*. New York: Dutton.

Ho, Mae-Wan. 1998. *Genetic Engineering: Dream or Nightmare?* New York: Continuum Publishing.

Inkamana, Lorna. 2002. "Snake Dreaming," painting #LI1. www.nanou.com.au/songlines.

IONS Noetic Sciences Review, Sausalito, Calif. (Generally helpful magazine.)

Johnson, John L., "Environmental Justice for All: Principles and Practices for Conflict Resolvers," *AcreSolution*, Summer 2002: 24ff.

Journal for Frontier Sciences at Temple University in Philadelphia. (Generally helpful magazine for understanding biophysics and medicine.)

Jung, Carl Gustav. 1924. "Kindertraume" [Childhood Dreams].

Unpublished manuscript of lectures given at the E.T.H. (Eidgenoische Technische Hochschule) in Zurich, Switzerland.

———. 1958. *Psychology and Religion: West and East, Vol. 11.*

———. 1960. "Synchronicity: An Acausal Connecting Principle." *The Structure and Dynamics of the Psyche: The Collected Works of C. G. Jung, Vol. 8.* Translated by R. F. C. Hull. Bollingen Series XX. London: Routledge.

———. 1968. *Psychology and Alchemy, Vol. 12.*

Kahn, Hazrat Inayat. 2001. *Sufi Message of Hazrat Inayat Khan.* (Sufi Message Series) New York: Hunter House.

Kaku, Michio. 1994. *Hyperspace: A Scientific Odyssey through Parallel Universes, Time Warps, and the Tenth Dimension.* New York: Anchor Books Doubleday.

Kircher, Athanasius. 1986. *Oedipus Aegyptiacus.* 1652/1986. Source: Thomas A.P. van Leeuwen, *The Skyward Trend of Thought.* Cambridge, Mass.: MIT Press.

Krishna, Gopi. 1971. *The Biological Basis of Religion and Genius,* with an introduction by Carl von Weizsacker, New York and London: Harper and Row.

Landau, L. D., and E. M. Lifshitz. 1999. *Statistical Physics,* 3rd ed. *Course of Theoretical Physics, Vol. 5.* Translated by J. B. Sykes and M. J. Kearsley. Oxford, UK: Butterworth-Heinemann.

Laszlo, Ervin. 1993. *The Creative Cosmos: A Unified Science of Matter, Life, and Mind.* Edinburgh: Floris Books.

Levin, Theodore, and Michael Edgerton. 1999, September. "The Throat Singers of Tuva." *Scientific American.* www.sciam.com/1999/0999issue/0999levin.html.

Leviton, Richard. 1992. "Landscape Mysteries and Healing Gaia: A Précis of Spiritual Geomancy." *West Coast Astrologer-Geomancer,* March, p. 15.

———. 2000. *Physician: Medicine and the Unsuspected Battle for Human Freedom.* Charlottesville, Va.: Hampton Roads.

————. 2002. *The Galaxy on Earth: A Traveler's Guide to the Planet's Visionary Geography.* Charlottesville, Va.: Hampton Roads.

Long, Derek A. 2001. *The Raman Effect: A Unified Treatment of the Theory of Raman Scattering by Molecules.* New York: John Wiley & Sons.

Lusseyran, Jacques. 1998. *And There Was Light: Autobiography of Jacques Lusseyran, Blind Hero of the French Resistance.* New York: Parabola Books.

McEvoy, J. P., and Oscar Zarate. 1999. *Quantum Theory for Beginners.* Cambridge, UK: Icon Books.

Menken, Dawn. 2002. *Speak Out! Talking About Love, Sex, and Eternity.* Tempe, Ariz.: New Falcon.

Mindell, Amy. 1994/2001. *Metaskills: the Spiritual Art of Therapy.* Tempe, Ariz.: New Falcon; Portland, Ore.: Lao Tse Press. laotse@e-z.net.

————. 1999. *Coma, A Healing Journey: A Guide for Family, Friends, and Helpers.* Portland, Ore.: Lao Tse Press. laotse@e-z.net.

————. 2002. *An Alternative to Therapy. A Few Basic Process Work Principles.* Zero Publications. (Available through Lao Tse Press. laotse@e-z.net.)

Mindell, Arnold. 1982. *Dreambody: The Body's Role in Revealing the Self.* Boston: Sigo Press.

————. 1984. *Working with the Dreaming Body.* London, England: Penguin-Arkana.

————. 1987. *Dreambody in Relationships.* New York and London: Penguin.

————. 1994. *Coma, Key to Awakening: Working with the Dreambody Near Death.* New York and London: Penguin-Arkana.

————. 1996. *The Shaman's Body: A New Shamanism for Transforming Health, Relationships, and Community.* San Francisco: HarperCollins.

———. 1997. *Sitting in the Fire: Large Group Transformation Through Diversity and Conflict*. Portland, Ore: Lao Tse Press. laotse@e-z.net.

———. 2000. *The Quantum Mind: The Edge between Physics and Psychology*. Portland Ore.: Lao Tse Press. laotse@e-z.net.

———. 2001. *Dreaming While Awake: Techniques for 24-Hour Lucid Dreaming*. Charlottesville, Va.: Hampton Roads.

———. 2002. *The Dreammaker's Apprentice: Using Heightened States of Consciousness to Interpret Dreams*. Charlottesville, Va.: Hampton Roads.

———. 2002. *The Deep Democracy of Open Forums: Practical Steps to Conflict Prevention and Resolution for the Family, Workplace, and World*. Charlottesville, Va.: Hampton Roads.

Morin, Pierre. 2002. *Rank and Salutogenesis: A Quantitative and Empirical Study of Self-Rated Health and Perceived Social Status*. Dissertation. Cincinnati: Union Institute.

Muktananda, Swami. 1994. *Kundalini: The Secret of Life*. South Fallsberg, N.Y.: Syda Foundation.

Nadeau, Robert, and Menas Kafatos. 1999. *The Non-Local Universe: The New Physics and Matters of the Mind*. New York: Oxford University Press.

New, Eldon. www.geocities.com/Athens/Acropolis/2606/superpos.htm.

North, Carolyn. 1997. *Death: The Experience of a Lifetime*. Berkeley, Calif.: Regent Press.

Pais, Abraham. 2000. *The Genius of Science*. London: Oxford University Press.

Peat, David F. 1990. *Einstein's Moon: Bell's Theorem and the Curious Quest for Quantum Reality*. Chicago: Contemporary Books.

Penrose, Roger. 1989. *The Emperor's New Mind*. London: Oxford University Press.

———. 1994. *Shadows of the Mind.* London: Oxford University Press.

Pert, Candice. 1999. *Molecules of Emotion.* New York: Simon and Schuster.

Pickover, Clifford A. 1999. *Surfing through Hyperspace: Understanding Higher Universes in Six Easy Lessons.* New York: Oxford University Press.

Price, Michael Clive. 2002. "The Everett FAQ." www.hedweb.com/everett/everett.htm.

Rawson, Philip, and Laszlo Legeza. 1973. *Tao: Eastern Philosophy of Time and Change.* New York: Avon Books.

Ray, Reginald. 2000. *Indestructible Truth: The Living Spirituality of Tibetan Buddhism.* London: Shambhala.

Reiss, Gary. 2001. *Changing Ourselves, Changing Our World.* Tempe, Ariz.: New Falcon.

Regis, Ed. 1995. *Nano: The Emerging Science of Nanotechnology.* New York: Little Brown.

Rinpoche, Sogyal. 1997. *The Tibetan Book of Living and Dying.* San Francisco: HarperCollins.

Rossi, Ernst. 2002. *The Psychobiology of Gene Expression: Neuroscience and Neurogenesis in Hypnosis and the Healing Arts.* New York: W. W. Norton.

Roth, Harold D. 1999. *Original Tao.* New York: Columbia University Press.

Rucker, Rudy. 1984. *The Fourth Dimension.* Boston: Houghton-Mifflin.

Sarfatti, Jack. 2001. "Post Quantum Physics." www.qedcorp.com/pcr/pcr/.

Schrödinger, Erwin. 1944. *What Is Life? With Mind and Matter and Autobiographical Sketches.* Cambridge, UK: Cambridge University Press.

Schupbach, Max. 2002. "Process Work." In S. Shannon, ed., *Handbook of Complimentary and Alternative Therapies in Mental Health.* New York: Academic Press.

Schwarz, Patricia. 2002. "Official Super String Website." www.super stringtheory.com/basics/index.html.

Sheldrake, Rupert. 1981. *A New Science of Life: The Hypothesis of Formative Causation*. Los Angeles: J. P. Tarcher.

———. 1988. *The Presence of the Past: Morphic Resonance and the Habits of Nature*. New York: Times Books.

———. 1990. *The Rebirth of Nature: The Greening of Science and God*. London and Sydney: Century.

———. 1997. "Part 1: Mind, Memory, and Archetype: Morphic Resonance and the Collective Unconscious" in *Psychological Perspectives*, vol. 18, no. 1, pp. 9–25, Fall 1997. Los Angeles: C. G. Jung Institute of Los Angeles.

———. 2002. "Sheldrake Online." www.sheldrake.org.

Sheldrake, Rupert, Ralph Abraham, and Terence McKenna. 1992. *Trialogues at the Edge of the West: Chaos, Creativity, and the Resacralization of the World*. Santa Fe, N.M.: Bear & Company Publishing.

Stargrove, Mitch. 2003. "Vital Systems: Integrative Medicine, Wellness, and the Healing Process." www.VitalSystems.org.

Strachan, Alan. 1993. "The Wisdom of the Dreaming Body: A Case Study of a Physical Symptom." *Journal of Process Oriented Psychology*, 5(2). Portland, Ore.: Lao Tse Press.

Sutton, Peter, et al., eds. 1989. *Dreamings: The Art of Aboriginal Australia*. New York: George Braziller.

Taber's Cyclopedic Medical Dictionary. 2001 Donald Venes, Clayton L. Thomas (eds). Clarence Wilbur Taber. Philadelphia: F.A. David Co.

Tompkins, Peter, and Christopher Bird. 1989. *The Secret Life of Plants*. New York: HarperCollins.

Von Franz, Marie Louise. 1978. *Time: Rhythm and Repose*. London: Thames and Hudson.

Von Neumann, John. 1932. *The Mathematical Foundations of Quantum Mechanics*. Princeton: Princeton University Press.

Wheeler, John Archibald, and Max Tegmark. 2001. "100 Years of Quantum Mysteries." *Scientific American,* vol. 284, no.1. pp. 68–75.

Wilhelm, Richard, trans. 1981. *I Ching*, or *Book of Changes*. Bollingen Series. Princeton, N.J.: Princeton University Press.

Wolf, Fred Alan. 1981. *Taking the Quantum Leap: The New Physics for Non-Scientists*. San Francisco: Harper & Row.

———. 1984. *Starwave: Mind, Consciousness, and Quantum Physics*. New York: Collier Books.

———. 1988. *Parallel Universe*. New York: Simon and Schuster.

Yi-Fu Tuan. 1993. *Passing Strange and Wonderful: Aesthetics, Nature, and Culture*. Washington, D.C.: Island Press.

Zohar, Danah. 1990. *The Quantum Self*. New York: William Morrow.

Index

Index

About the Author

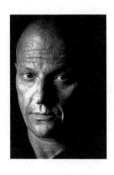

ARNOLD MINDELL, Ph.D., is known worldwide for his innovative synthesis of dreams and bodywork, Jungian therapy and group process, quantum physics, and conflict resolution. Dr. Mindell travels widely, holding workshops and making frequent appearances on television and radio. He lives in Portland, Oregon.

Hampton Roads Publishing Company

. . . for the evolving human spirit

Hampton Roads Publishing Company
publishes books on a variety of subjects,
including metaphysics, health,
visionary fiction, and other related topics.

For a copy of our latest catalog, call toll-free
(800) 766-8009, or send your name and address to:

Hampton Roads Publishing Company, Inc.
1125 Stoney Ridge Road
Charlottesville, VA 22902

e-mail: hrpc@hrpub.com
www.hrpub.com